KEYS TO
HEALTHY COMMUNICATION:
AUTHENTICITY,
EMPATHY,
EMPOWERMENT

Bobby R. Patton, Ph.D.

Rusalyn H. Andrews, Ph.D.

Jennifer Page Daily, M.D.

Tridox Publishing

LAWRENCE, KANSAS

2022

Paperback ISBN: 9780578317861

eBook ISBN: 9780578317878

PRINTED IN THE UNITED STATES OF AMERICA

Table of Contents

Preface

In January of 2020 the World Health Organization (WHO) reported the outbreak of a new coronavirus , SARS-CoV-2, spreading from China to other countries around the world. The WHO and public health authorities in many countries began acting to contain the outbreak. Two months later, as the disease spread rapidly from country to country with attendant stress and deaths mounting, the WHO made the assessment to characterize COVID-19 as a PANDEMIC.

The U.S. was one of the countries particularly vulnerable to this new virus. Despite continuing advances in medical research and vast economic expenditures, U.S. health had been declining for several years in comparison to other advanced nations and its own past. Life expectancy in the U.S. dropped for the fifth year in a row in 2020. As reported by the Center for Disease Control, this downward trend was the first sustained lifespan decline in the U.S. since World War I. Contributing to this decline, in addition to medical and nutritional issues, were greater reliance on addictive drugs, increased number of suicides, and increased rates of depression, stress, anger issues, and toxic relationships . The health of U.S. society was also impacted by ever widening political differences, including international tensions, and a growing absence of trust. These stresses resulted in polarized disagreements over core values, including whether access to public health care is a "right" or a "privilege."

Authors Bobby Patton, Rusalyn Andrews, and Jennifer Daily first met in early 2017 to share concerns over the many factors influencing the nation's alarmingly declining health. After extended discussions, they realized that the choices made in communication, often reflexively and habitually, make a difference in whether the results are healthy or unhealthy. They concluded it was time to create a book that identifies detrimental communication practices associated with unhealthy outcomes and suggests healthy communication alternatives.

The authors come from diverse backgrounds. Their ages span three generations; their academic resumes differ, and their life experiences both professionally and personally are varied. Bobby R. Patton (Ph.D., University of Kansas, 1966) has been a communication scholar, a professor and an administrator at four major public universities, including serving as President at the University of Central Missouri. He has co-authored sixteen highly regarded college textbooks in the area of interpersonal communication and decision making. In 2021 he received the Albert Nelson Marquis Lifetime Achievement Award. Rusalyn H. Andrews (Ph.D., Southern Illinois University, Carbondale, 1989) is a professor emeritus of Cottey College, a private women's liberal arts institution. She has taught courses in communication, theatre, and women, gender and sexuality studies. She has rich international educational experiences, including a Fulbright Award to do research in Russia, and specialized training in Deaf Culture. Jennifer Page Daily, (M.D.,

University of Nevada, 2007), the youngest member of the team, is a Board-Certified Family Practice Physician with a Certificate of Added Qualification in Primary Care Sports Medicine. She is an Associate Professor at the University of Louisville in the Department of Family and Geriatric Medicine. She serves as a course director for the Introduction to Clinical Medicine, a pre-clinical course for all university medical students. In 2018, Dr. Daily was the recipient of the Department's Excellence in Teaching Award and Outstanding Faculty Award. She also was named a 2018 Inspirational Physician by the American Medical Association Women Physicians Section. In 2020 she received the Exemplary Teaching Award from the Kentucky Academy of Family Physicians, and in 2021 she was named a member of Alpha Omega Alpha National Honor Medical Society.

The humanistic approach and conceptual framework expressed in this book are directly attributable to the late Carl Rogers (1902-1987). Bobby Patton, who served for a time on his staff at The Center for Study of the Person in La Jolla, California, recalls asking Rogers why these concepts were not being shared with a larger audience. Rogers' thoughtful response was, "We have to begin somewhere." Your authors are attempting to take the next step by citing the best information on healthy communication from reliable research. They also base their framework on a process perspective that recognizes the interdependence and relatedness of all things. People are in a continual process of making choices that result in their actions. Those actions have consequences, and the decisions made lead to healthy or unhealthy outcomes. The writing is based on the most current information available, recognizing that the body of research grows daily.

The authors recognize and emphasize the importance of interpersonal communication to individual health. Interpersonal communication is the basis for a person's significant relationships, social interactions, and emotions toward others; choices are made when to terminate, deepen, or merely tolerate a relationship. The importance of our social lives has been repeatedly studied by psychologists, sociologists, health professionals and behavioral scientists. We believe that three concepts determine health and successful development of interpersonal relationships. These concepts are truly keys to healthy communication, and include not only behaviors, but also attitudes, feelings and commitment to healthy choices:

1. Authenticity—involves honesty, trust, truth, openness and reliability. Authentic behavior is likely to be met in kind and result in good will and reciprocated trust.

2. Empathy—capacity to understand, feel, and accept the other. Not only should "we walk in the other's shoes," we must think and feel as they do to fully understand, feel and engage.

3. Empowerment—freedom from external power, control and manipulation; freedom to make decisions and act as one chooses guided by legal and ethical principles .

The framework of this book will explore these concepts in depth through the context of:

      1. Personal Health—all aspects of mental and physical health.

      2. Relational Health—how people relate to partners, friends, family, work associates and even strangers.

      3. Societal Health—the communication practices that can affect people's collective future.

This book was completed late in 2021 as the country was adjusting to major changes brought on by the Biden presidency and the widespread disbursement of three successful COVID-19 vaccines. When over half of the U.S. population became protected by the vaccine, optimism returned for a brief time. On July 4, Americans celebrated the holidays with parties, trips to the beach, and family gatherings. The new Delta variant, a more contagious form of the virus, took advantage of this opportunity, and the virus surged again.

The five years spent preparing this book obviously included the COVID-19 pandemic as it spread across the globe. The authors began their project with the intent to avoid politics, but the crisis became political from the outset. While the authors did not know each other's political beliefs at the beginning of the project, they were united in their belief in truth and science based on verifiable evidence. They utilized consensus to maintain a shared view of reality. Sadly, by the end of 2021, over 800,000 Americans had died from the COVID-19 virus.

Acknowledgements

This book was made possible by the assistance and support of many people. Joanne Haugland provided typing and additional assistance while the authors worked in Chandler, AZ. In Kansas, Nancy Harmony served as the copy editor. The University of Kansas Office of Digital and Media Services, especially Pam LeRow and Eric Bader, provided valuable assistance in the lay-out and formatting of the book. Eleanor Patton served as copy editor and constructive critic. Rusalyn Andrews acknowledges the support of her children, Sarah Andrews-Weiss and Wil Weiss, her daughter-in-law Xanda Weiss, and the newest member of the family, her grandson Jon. Jennifer Page Daily values the help and support of her husband, Mark Daily, the excused absences by her sons, Lincoln and Harrison, and the early feedback from her parents, Paul and Jeanne Page. We thank Sarah Cooper for typing format help, Vincent LaVallee of el Consulting LLC for essential technical support, and Sarah Andrews Weiss for copy editing.

The authors acknowledge their debt to Carl Rogers for providing the theoretical grounding for this work and, additionally, Kim Giffin (trust), Sidney M. Jourard (humanistic psychology), Daniel Goleman (neuroscience; multiple intelligence), Steven Pinker (cognitive psychology and human nature), Michael Marmot (health determinants), and Jonathan Page (neuroscience and cognitive control) as well as numerous others who will be noted in the endnotes to each chapter.

We are indebted to Beth Berg and Mark Osborn, MD, who read drafts of the manuscript and offered invaluable advice. We appreciate the cartoons created by a late friend, Charles Barsotti. Peter Riva, our agent, has provided thoughtful guidance to the manuscript.

Chapter 1 - A Perspective of Health and Wellness

This book was being written as the COVID-19 pandemic exploded around the world. By experiencing such a health crisis in the process of writing about strategies for a healthier future, we became more convinced than ever that this book can help you understand and improve your health and well-being. The concepts and practices described here encompass and also transcend this crisis, and provide guidance for improving our health and building the world that we envision for our collective futures.

This pandemic focused attention on world health as never before, exposing problems both within and among countries struggling with divergent points of view, distrust, fear, and the threat of violence. It also generated vivid public examples of social divisions and the inability of leaders to communicate clearly and support good health practices. The U.S. will have a collective memory of this crisis and its effects.

Your quality of life is linked directly to your personal health (physical health, mental/emotional health, and spiritual health), relational health, and societal health. In turn, the quality of your health is directly linked to communication behaviors. Some communication enhances life and the personal health of the people involved; other interactions are destructive. For example, recent research in social neuroscience has demonstrated that when an individual is performing a task, support from a loved one not only feels good, but also calms the areas of the brain that produce stress hormones detrimental to your health. We have chosen to label communication behaviors that support health in its many forms as "healthy communication," and conversely, communication that is detrimental to health as "unhealthy communication."

While "health" is a term that is widely used and understood, even the medical profession is unable to agree upon an exact definition. Consider for a moment the differences between "illness" and "wellness." A person may feel well but have a blocked coronary artery, while another person may have extreme back pain, but no evidence of muscle or disc damage. A person carrying the coronavirus may have no detectable symptoms but be contagious. Who is "sick" and who is "well"?

The **World Health Organization** defines health as the following: **A state of complete physical, mental and social well-being...Not merely the absence of disease or infirmity...That leads to a socially and economically productive life.** This widely accepted definition from the WHO suggests that it is possible to have a healthy body, mind, spirit, and society. Health is the ability to perform effectively, particularly in terms of family and work. The goal is a wellness that encompasses the entire person, rather than just a lack of physical pain or disease. Health promotion consists of the development of lifestyle habits which healthy individuals and communities can adopt to maintain and enhance their state of well-being.

Personal Health

The WHO definition of health views personal health from three perspectives: Physical, Mental and Spiritual. Here is a brief overview of each.

Physical Health

Your goal is to have a healthy body. Many conditions are outside your control, such as genetic defects, injuries, and certain diseases, but you still can optimize your personal health through the choices you make. As an example, consider the health of your teeth and gums that are affected by your patterns of dental hygiene. Fortunately, the work of the National Human Genome Research Institute now allows us to identify certain problematic genes and take precautionary measures to reduce their impact on our health.

A single poor choice can affect aspects of your health throughout your lifetime, but frequently your health patterns are affected by recurring choices that forge habitual patterns in your health practices. These unconscious choices may include such things as diet and nutrition, type and amount of exercise or other physical activity, and your choice of friends and partners. Involvement with social networks can affect such behaviors as smoking, drinking alcohol, using drugs, or how much food you consume. They all have an impact on your well-being.

Mental Health

A healthy mind is characterized by the absence of, or the management of, such mental disorders as depression, anxiety, eating disorders, bipolar disorders, and personality disorders. Millions of people throughout the world are affected by such disorders. Even more striking is the fact that the vast majority of people have never undergone a mental health evaluation. As Chris Segrin, communication professor at the University of Arizona, has noted:

> Consider for example, the results of recent epidemiological investigations indicating that in any given year 28 percent of the adults in the United States have some form of psychological disorder and that 48 percent of the U.S. population will have a diagnosable psychological disorder at some time in their lives. Given the pervasiveness of mental health problems in society, it is likely that most people will have a relationship (be it romantic, family, friendly, occupational, or professional) with someone suffering from a mental health problem and/or will experience a mental health problem themselves.[1]

The current COVID-19 epidemic has spurred fear on a societal level. On an individual level, anxiety may be exacerbated and lead to non-specific mental issues such as mood problems, sleep issues, phobia-like behavior, panic, and psychosis-like symptoms. Mental health authorities urge their colleagues to use sound informational control practices and help their communities maintain civil, courteous and rational communication.[2]

Adverse Childhood Experiences, or ACEs, are now recognized by the Centers for Disease Control and Prevention as an important public health issue. Childhood experiences, both positive and negative, have a tremendous impact on future violence, victimization and perpetration, and lifelong health.[3] Only recently have routine pediatric screenings been able to identify early signs of neurodevelopmental disorders. Some medical practices are now asking about and documenting ACE scores to identify stressors in a child's home. The CDC-Kaiser ACE Study demonstrated that Adverse Childhood Experiences contributes to disrupted neurodevelopment, which leads to social, emotional and cognitive impairment. If interventions are not made, a child or teenager is more likely to adopt unhealthy and high-risk behaviors that can lead to disease, disability, social problems, and premature death.

The teenage years are a critical time in the development of human minds and brains. The brain does not fully mature until late adolescence and early adulthood, when the prefrontal cortex undergoes the final stages of building and organization. This area has been shown to control impulses, judgments, rational thinking, and moral reasoning. Some acts of irrational and impulsive behavior may be attributable to immaturity.[4]

During the stress and disrupted lifestyles created by the COVID-19 epidemic, children often sought more attention and demanded more parental time. Parents were encouraged to discuss the situation with their children in an honest and age-appropriate way. If children had concerns, parents were advised to address them. During unusual times, children more closely observe adult behavior and emotions, for cues on how to react and manage their own.

Spiritual Health

As we have noted, the World Health Organization (WHO) includes spiritual health as a component that contributes to one's well-being. This topic is the least discussed because of its closeness to religion. However, if high levels of total wellness cannot be achieved without a balance of all of the dimensions – mind, body, and spirit – spirit must be included. This discussion is not from any single religious perspective or mystical orientation; rather, it is an attempt to better understand from a humanistic perspective, what spiritual health is and how it interacts with other dimensions of health.

Spiritual health seems to provide a life purpose and meaning to existence;[5] it provides a sense of wholeness in life based upon a consistent set of principles, ethics, and values.[6] Such beliefs provide the basis for appreciation of beauty and a sense of connectedness to others; they provide the basis for feelings of love, joy, hope, and fulfillment.[7]

Spiritually healthy individuals seem to have a coherent system of beliefs that explain their reality. These beliefs do not have to be religious, but they do answer questions such as: "Why am I here?"; "What provides meaning and fulfillment to my life?"; "How can I achieve happiness and satisfaction?" In answering these questions, each of us feels a greater sense of purpose and meaning for our existence, and a path toward personal fulfillment. This spiritual health perspective provides a person with a congruent set of moral values, beliefs and guides for conduct that permit people to feel good about themselves. Discussions of spirituality typically include such concepts as compassion, selflessness, honesty, integrity, and connectedness with others.[8] Such concepts have been shown to be instrumental to mental and physical health. Consider for a moment the unhealthy alternatives. For example, the opposite of selflessness would be self-gratification. Individuals who are so inclined to indulge in pleasure-seeking behavior are more prone to addictions, and feelings of emptiness.[9]

Spiritual health manifests itself in interpersonal communication. Healthy individuals communicate with honesty, integrity, trust, compassion, and a genuine concern for others . A direct correlation exists between the need for love and acceptance and spiritual health. As with physical and mental health, this dimension of health is nurtured during infancy and childhood within the context of a loving family. A perception of love and acceptance is the prerequisite to self-esteem. This self-esteem is intrinsic to the views of reality, values and ethics that are modeled to each of us early in our lives. People with healthy spirits find beauty and connectedness in life, tolerance and acceptance of others, and a fuller acceptance of self.[10]

Spiritual health is closely intertwined with mental and physical health. Spiritual health provides an individual with life purpose and an ultimate meaning to life; it is the basis for principles, values, and ethics, as well as feelings of love, peace, hope and fulfillment. Healthy spirit is thus identified by healthy communication.[11]

Relational Health

In addition to the three components of personal health as defined by the World Health Organization, relational health and societal health also heavily impact people's well-being.

A large body of literature documents the linkage between our social relationships and physical health. Epidemiological studies have shown connections between a lack of social support and increased risk of disease and reduced length of life.[12] The CDC-Kaiser ACE Study also demonstrated this relationship, and its impact on morbidity and mortality.

Bert N. Uchino, a professor of psychology at the University of Utah, has suggested four categories of social support:

- **Emotional** – expressions of caring and validation from someone who makes you feel better because they truly listen to you.
- **Informational** – advice and guidance from someone you trust and respect.
- **Tangible** – support in the form of material aid, such as money or services.
- **Belonging** – togetherness involving shared social activities; the sheer joy of friends being together and enjoying time with each other.[13]

The theoretical links between social relationships and well-being are relatively straightforward; they start with the premise that relationship partners provide resources that one individual cannot acquire on his or her own. Each of us has limited skills, knowledge, information, strength, and energy.[14]

Just as healthy communication is a major contributor to emotional well-being, it is also crucial to your positive relationship experiences and, thus, your physical health. As Michael Argyle has stated: "social relationships are a major source of happiness, relief from distress and health".[15]

The Mayo Clinic points out that chronic stressful life situations can increase the risk of developing depression. Depression has become such a common health problem that in January 2016, the U.S. Prevention Services Task Force, which advises the federal government on health, recommended that primary care doctors screen all adults for depression. Major depression disorder, a severe type of depression, is the leading cause of disability in the U.S., according to the task force. Nearly 7 percent of American adults, or about 16 million people, had at least one "major depression episode" in 2020 according to the National Alliance on Mental Illness. Depression can be life-threatening. More than 50,000 Americans commit suicide each year, about 90 percent related to mental illness. A 2015 study in the *Journal of Clinical Psychiatry* estimated that depression costs the U.S. $210 billion a year, with 40 percent related directly to depression and the rest to indirect costs such as lost productivity.[16]

The insurance company Blue Cross-Blue Shield released a report on May 14, 2018 which showed that major depression among Americans was on the rise. The report found that the number of people suffering from depression jumped 33 percent from 2013 through 2016. Millennials and teenagers have experienced even faster rates of depression – up to 47 percent for millennials and 63 percent for teenagers.[17] These rates have continued to rise during the pandemic.

A major factor for the rapid rise in the depression rate for teens appears to be the increased amount of time using media screens. Researchers at San Diego State and Florida State Universities found that nearly half of teens who spent five or more hours a day in front of screens experienced "thoughts of suicide or prolonged periods of hopelessness or sadness."[18]

The most common sources of stress identified by individuals are: other people, relationships, and interactions with others. Interpersonal communication can create and promote stress or it can buffer and relieve stress. Dr. Teresa Seeman has researched in detail how we can be positively or negatively impacted by our social interactions. After exhaustive study, she concluded: "Humans appear to be exquisitely responsive to our social relationships – not only cognitively and emotionally, but physiologically as well – both as recipients and purveyors of positive and/or negative communication."[19]

During the pandemic of 2020, the isolation required yielded the expected results. Families that practiced healthy communication experienced relatively pleasant passage of time. For many, however, the protocol of bleach wipes and masks were insignificant compared to the daily task of disinfecting unhealthy interactions. Toxic relationships fueled by enforced close proximity produced increased stress, conflict and abusive behaviors. While most crimes showed significant decline due to limited interaction, fraud, domestic violence and abuse within families spiked.

Societal Health

The definition of "healthy society" used in this book derives from the authors' diverse academic backgrounds as a social scientist, humanities scholar, and medical professional and researcher. A healthy society as used in this book is defined as the following: a conglomerate of interdependent contributing citizens who create and endow their government with deserved trust and the power necessary to peacefully coordinate and meet the needs of its citizenry, while peacefully co-existing with other societies.

Dr. Steven A. Schroeder wrote an influential article in 2007 for *The New England Journal of Medicine* entitled, "We Can Do Better in Improving the Health of the American People." He asks why it is that while the U.S. spends more on health care than any other nation in the world, it ranks poorly on nearly every measure of health status. One measure where we exceeded others was in life expectancy, a category that we led every year until 2016.

Schroeder states that health is influenced by five "domains" – genetics, social circumstances, environmental exposure, behavioral patterns, and health care. He further points out that our behaviors have a larger impact in determining our health than any other category. "The deaths lie in personal behavior. In fact, behavioral causes accounted for nearly 40 percent of all deaths in the United States."[20] The proportional contributions to premature death in 2007, categorized by Schroeder's domains, were as follows: environmental exposure – 5 percent, health care – 10 percent, social circumstances – 15 percent, genetic predisposition – 30 percent and behavioral patterns – 40 percent.[21]

Good social policies impact behavioral choices in a positive way. Seat belt laws have saved lives. Tobacco labelling and increased taxation have deterred use. Nutritional labelling of foods allows healthy dietary choices. Taxation, housing, education, and transportation have important health consequences.

Health differences related to socio-economic status were further magnified during the COVID-19 pandemic. African Americans died at an alarmingly higher rate than others. In Louisiana, for example, African Americans comprised 33 percent of the population, but accounted for 70 percent of COVID-19 deaths . The disparity can be partially attributable to economic disparities that affect diet, insurance availability, housing, and access to medical help.

Societies responded in various ways to the pandemic of 2020. The Chinese government moved psychiatrists to Wuhan during the first stage of self-quarantine. No comparable measures were initiated by our federal government. While both the federal and local governments (some alarmingly slower than others) responded to the spread of the coronavirus in a range of critical ways, acknowledgement of mental illness was cursory. The exception was Governor Andrew Cuomo of New York, who enlisted more than 8,000 mental health providers to help New Yorkers in distress.

The Health Continuum

Your physical health, mental and emotional health, relationship health, and the health of your society are all interrelated. If you were asked to describe your current state of health, all of these elements would be germane. Your health is not an absolute state, and being healthy does not mean that you will never be sick.

Physical health is the way your body parts and systems work together. You need the ability to cope with the stresses of daily life with strength and energy. To maintain your physical health, you need good nutrition, sufficient sleep and rest, and physical activity. You must practice good hygiene to prevent disease, and get regular medical checkups, treatments and immunizations. You should make choices to try to avoid contagious diseases and dangerous environments and behaviors, as well as resisting known harmful agents such as tobacco and narcotics.

Your mental and emotional health includes your feelings about yourself, how well you relate to others, and how well you meet the demands of daily life. A person with good emotional health is in touch with his or her feelings and expresses them appropriately. The problems and frustrations of life are able to be handled without feeling overwhelmed.

Your relationship health involves the way you get along with others, particularly intimate others. You have the ability to make and keep friends, to work and socialize in cooperative ways. You seek and lend support as needed, share respect, and care for yourself and others.

You contribute to, and are influenced by, the health and well-being of society. When members of a society act in honest, truthful and trusting ways, they elicit complementary responses. Manipulation, deceit, and dishonesty perpetrate the same negative behaviors. The health of society is determined by the choices of its members.

A person with a balanced life can be said to have a high degree of wellness, good health, and an overall state of well-being. Achieving excellent health or wellness is a lifelong commitment to physical, mental/emotional, relational, and societal health. You must live each day making decisions based on healthful attitudes and healthy communications.

As a work in process, your health is dynamic. You are constantly being bombarded with messages from social media and television, as well as pressures from others that can impact your health. The fact that your health is dynamic means that it fluctuates along a *continuum* (as shown in Figure 1.1). Like a yardstick, there are different points where your health can be located at any given time. Picture such a continuum as a line representing all possible degrees of health. The far-left end of the line represents the total absence of health: death. On the far-right end is the highest possible level of wellness or maximum well-being. The center point of the line represents a lack of disease, freedom from aches and pains and moderate energy. From day to day, you may experience different levels of health in each category. Sudden changes may occur, or shifts may be gradual.

Decide where you presently would place yourself along each of the four lines. Determine where you need change. You may recognize areas of your own wellness continuum that can be improved. This book explains how your interpersonal communication behaviors play a key role in your mental, physical and spiritual health. As you adopt the healthier options this book offers you, you will be rewarded by a healthier and happier life.

Figure 1.1: The Personal Health Continuum

Minimal State of Health	———————	Mid-Point	———————	Optimum State of Health

Physical Health

| Chronic disorders
Chronic pain
Loss of ability/bodily control | Aches, pains &
lack of energy | Wellness fluctuates as
body naturally grows,
guards, & maintains itself | Consciously
maintains own
well-being | High energy
Temporary informative pain
Regenerative growth |

Mental/Emotional Health

| Mentally
disturbed | Inappropriate
responses to stress &
life situations
Anger & resentment | Healthy & unhealthy
survival strategies | Realistic perceptions
Positive attitudes | Ability to solve
personal
problems |

Relational Health

| Inability to sustain
meaningful
relationships | One-sided
manipulation
Hides true self | Rigidity in patterns
of behavior | Honest & open
Shows care &
empathy | Sustained loving
relationships
Allow personal &
relational growth |

Societal Health

| War & fear | Hatred & distrust
Lies & deception | Precarious
balance
Uncertainty | Trust & mutual
caring
Conflict resolution | Peace |

Just between Us

Do a self-inventory of your personal health on the seven topics listed below and discuss with a spouse or trusted other. Identify areas for improvement.

1. Sufficient sleep of high quality (8-9 hours).
2. A nutritionally balanced diet.
3. Appropriate exercise per week.
4. Appropriate safety practices such as wearing seat belts, protective gear, and avoidance of risky behaviors.
5. Avoidance of tobacco, drugs, and excessive alcohol.
6. Appropriate social support networks. Consider family, friends, and members of groups such as church and clubs.
7. Access to current and reliable health information.

Personal Reflections

1. How much do you know about your heredity? Talk with older relatives regarding the health and recurring problems in your family. Consult your medical provider regarding whether medical DNA testing would be of help in determining your own physical health strategies, family planning, or the way you raise your children.

2. Consider your physical environment. Do you experience stress or feel threatened for your safety? Do you feel that your living conditions are clean, safe, and free from health risks?

In the next chapter we will explore the inextricable connections between your health and your communication practices.

Chapter 2 - The Importance of Communication to Health

If you were asked to name the qualities you value most in your life, you might include good health, personal satisfactions and achievements, and treasured relationships. Seldom do you consider that communication is essential to acquiring and maintaining all these things you value.

In recent years, a primary focus of society has been on the health and well-being of all citizens: promoting health care, cessation of smoking, proper diets, exercise, and access to medical care. Yet, rarely has the discussion included discoveries of communication scholars, sociologists, psychologists, and neurologists regarding the unmistakable link between the quality of health and the quality of communication. That's the connection the authors of this book, want to discuss with you in this chapter.

Communication is basic to all human existence. From the first cry of a new-born to the whispered farewells of a near-death person, communication is intrinsic to all phases of human life. In fact, it is safe to say that communication is the true sign of life. When the body stops communicating, stops sending signs such as a detectable pulse, we determine that death has occurred. Social scientists have determined that whenever you are in the presence of another, some form of communicating is occurring. To ignore the other person actually sends a loud and clear message.

In the early 1960's, psychiatrist Jurgen Ruesch proposed that communication was an indicator of health. He regarded the mentally ill as persons who are deficient in skills necessary to fully communicate with other people. In other words, those with mental illness lack the ability to transmit thoughts and feelings, to monitor their own messages sent, and to understand meanings intended by others. By calling attention to the role played by communication in the attainment, indication, and maintenance of health, Ruesch opened the way to important areas of research, including how failure to communicate certain aspects of one's experience can seriously impair health, whereas frank and open communication makes possible the development of love and mutual growth.[22]

Think about your recent interactions. Are there some people who always seem to cause your blood pressure to rise? How does your body respond to stress and situations of conflict? Do you have friends who always make you feel relaxed and in a better mood? Advances in neuroscience have demonstrated that physical and mental health are invariably affected by the quality of communication we have with those surrounding us.

The world is constantly changing, and each change affects what comes next. Recognizing process helps people identify causes and effects and the interrelatedness of all occurrences, events, and experiences. What happens is not random; what happens is irreversible and in turn, sets other changes in motion .

In communication, a word spoken cannot be taken back. The concept of process provides a foundation for connections between communication and health.

Categories of Human Communication

Human communication takes many forms (written, spoken, nonverbal) and is both conscious and unconscious. Identifying and understanding the various forms are important because they help you to control the messages that you send, and how you respond to messages received. Humans have more choices in communication behavior than are realized. As unconscious communication actions become conscious, you are better able to control your communication in ways that can improve your health.

Most of you are born with all the tools you need to make good human contact, although some people have not found them or discovered how to use them. You need to understand how the tools work, how and when to use them, and the communication choices that are available to you. Once you understand these universal human tools, you can decide which ones will help with your health needs, and then work on developing those particular ones.

The authors find it helpful to distinguish between categories of human communication for discussion purposes.

INTRAPERSONAL COMMUNICATION is the most personal kind of communication occurring inside an individual. It includes thoughts, debates with oneself, and private decision making. Some medical professionals include intrapersonal communication methods as part of a patient's treatment for cancer (such as guided imagery and positive meditation), and note its positive effect on recovery. [23] Professionals can also teach patients how to lower blood pressure and respiratory rate through meditation and mindfulness practices. Intrapersonal communication comprises the internal processes involved in making decisions and taking action. Cartoonists have depicted the intrapersonal communication process by showing an angel on one shoulder debating with a devil on the other. Intrapersonal communication is the most common kind of communication, providing the foundation for all other communication. Signals are going continuously from all parts of your body to your brain. A mild stomach discomfort may suggest that you are hungry, or that you have overeaten. Intrapersonal communication thus refers to all the communication that transpires inside a person.

Other forms of intrapersonal communication include the perceptual notes you make, and the rationalizations and attitudes that determine overt behaviors. Basic to all levels of communication is a developed consciousness of self. As psychologist Rollo May observed:

> The capacity for consciousness of ourselves gives us the ability
> to see ourselves as others see us and to have empathy with others.
> It underlines our remarkable capacity to transport ourselves into

someone else's parlor where we will be, in reality next week, and then an imagination to think and plan how we will act. And it enables us to imagine ourselves in someone else's place, and to ask how we would feel and what we would do if we were this other person. No matter how poorly we use or fail to use or even abuse these capacities, they are the rudiments of our ability to love our neighbor, to have ethical sensitivity, to see truth, to create beauty, to devote ourselves to ideals, and to die for them if need be.[24]

May goes on to develop the thesis that fulfilling these potentials is the key to truly becoming a person. Intrapersonal communication allows people to be self-aware. In an ongoing monologue, you compare the person you wish to be to the person you believe you are. You determine what you will share of yourselves and what you will keep hidden. You develop attitudes about yourself and the world, making judgments that affect your behaviors, your emotions and very often your health. The ways that you shape these intrapersonal monologues shape your perceptions of everything, including your behaviors. Ultimately, they affect who you are, the value you place on yourself, your relationships, and your society.

Consider the "little voice in your head" that coaches you to succeed or discourages you as you attempt to achieve large and small goals. Heed the encouraging voice and challenge the negative one. Recurring issues and concerns regarding your intrapersonal communication should be discussed with a mental health professional.

IMPERSONAL COMMUNICATION occurs between people when they make no effort to recognize each other as unique individuals. The other person is treated not as an individual but as an interchangeable component. Impersonal communication occurs when you relate to others because they fill a role or satisfy an immediate need. You do not differentiate or treat the other person in any way unique or special. These routine types of communication occur when you do not wish to exert time or energy to build a relationship. In a restaurant, for example, you interact with the waiter who is fulfilling his or her role in meeting your needs. You may exchange information with no need to establish a continuing relationship.

Impersonal communication is based on functionality and good sense. You interact with many people as needed to fulfill your employment obligations and common courtesy. These interactions are usually too limited to form lasting relationships.

Impersonal communication seeks payoffs that have little to do with the people involved. When planning to purchase a television, you may work with the salesperson to find one best suited to your needs. Out of necessity, you interact in impersonal ways frequently. At its best, impersonal communication helps to efficiently expedite everyday tasks.

14

At its worst, impersonal communication involves treating other people as objects. You may interact with others as stereotypes or fulfill roles that do not permit you to communicate with people as distinct individuals. During the height of the COVID-19 pandemic, people tended to avoid individuals with whom they might otherwise interact impersonally. They sought to avoid interactions that had a potential of spreading disease by having groceries delivered to their cars and doors by nameless, masked individuals with whom there was little conversation. Classes and meetings were held on-line to provide distance. People stopped eating out, congregating, and meeting with people. People were seen as potential sources of infection and impersonal threats. In some circumstances, such actions are cruel and dysfunctional. While you may choose to dismiss abruptly a phone solicitor, you certainly do not want to automatically treat others as objects. Your co-workers, classmates, and certainly members of your family deserve to be treated with respect as individuals. Many horrific acts have been perpetrated on individuals who were perceived impersonally. Such acts are occurring right now in unhealthy relationships and unhealthy societies.

INTERPERSONAL COMMUNICATION is differentiated from impersonal communication by the choices made by the people involved. They are consciously aware of one another, and a relationship exists in some form. The conversation is unique with each party adapting to the other. There is spontaneity, expression of feelings, and a genuine attempt to share common meanings; levels of empathy are explicit. This type of communication establishes the basis for on-going deeper relationships.

Whenever people choose to engage in interpersonal communication, they take at least partial responsibility for how the other person responds and for the outcome of the communication. True interpersonal communication occurs with the following characteristics:

1. The transactional nature of interpersonal communication involves the influence each communicator exerts on the other. In other words, interpersonal communication isn't something done to others, but rather it's something that requires involvement of all participants. Interpersonal communication does not allow an "opt out." If your mind wanders from what your friend is saying, or you daydream rather than listen, the communication has been terminated. Communication may be either intentional or unintentional, but it is dependent upon the mutual needs of the people who wish to engage, promote mutual understanding, and participate in a relationship.

2. You communicate by translating thoughts of objects, actions and concepts into coded messages . As you attribute meaning to the words and behaviors of another person, you are inferring, with a varying degree of probability, what is going on inside that other individual. You attach meanings to behaviors that may or may not be valid. You cannot read

another person's mind, so you must settle for imperfect understanding.

3. Interpersonal communication is unique and irreversible. This characteristic means that true interpersonal communication has never happened before in the same fashion, and will never be repeated because the participants, the context, and the relational needs will never be the same. A single ill-chosen message may disrupt a relationship. Just as a clever lawyer knows that "to strike from the record" does not erase the impression made on a jury, you cannot take back your words or actions after the impact has been felt. Interpersonal communication has power and consequences.

4. Interpersonal communication establishes and defines the nature of the relationship between the people involved. Your interpersonal communication not only conveys information but, at the same time, sends a message concerning the relationship between the communicants. How you see and feel about yourself, and how you see and feel about others, are communicated by your manner, tone of voice, posture, eye contact, and other nonverbal means, as well as the words used. You look for clues about how the other person feels about you, who will have the most power in the relationship, and how involved the other party will be with you. Uncertainty regarding the other person's feelings and behaviors (and your own) are reduced as you get to know one another. These patterns of communication tend to be reciprocal. If you are friendly, I'll be friendly and vice-versa.

The idea here is that to be healthy people, to have healthy relationships, and to participate in healthy societies, you must assume responsibility for the communication that occurs with those you deem important enough to build enduring interpersonal relationships.

Social Media and Relationships

Interpersonal Relationships were challenged by the extreme shifts in daily behaviors imposed by COVID-19. Loved ones found themselves either separated or tightly sequestered. Some individuals lost loved ones without the opportunity to provide comfort, say goodbye, or even grieve. Face-to-face interpersonal interactions were replaced with creative solutions. Birthday parties were replaced with drive-by well-wishers. Phones and social media provided connectedness for those in need of interpersonal contact.

Social media can either enhance or diminish interpersonal relationships. We can use texts, phone calls, e-mails, virtual video calls, social media entries, blogs, and letters to enhance our relationships, sometimes saying and revealing information that we might not share in person. We can reflect, take our time choosing just the right words, and edit what we present on-line. We can review recorded words or responses, and withhold unflattering information.

Free from the restraints of spontaneous nonverbal communication, unscrupulous communicators can more successfully lie or present themselves untruthfully on line. While social media allows review, entries are hard to "erase." It's difficult to convince others we have changed when evidence of bad behavior continues to be available on-line. Users can overlook the fact that they are responding to other human beings and feel emboldened to post insensitive comments anonymously. These impersonal responses can be harsher than those delivered in person. Tactless comments, harsh criticism, harassment and cyber-bullying are too common.

Information on-line makes it easy to connect with people, but just as easy to stalk, cyber-stalk or harass. More than six months after the 2020 U. S. presidential election, election officials from Georgia and volunteers and their family members received death threats for not taking action to change presidential election results. Cyberbullying has been linked to such negative health conditions as withdrawal from society , depression, psychosomatic pain, drug and alcohol abuse, and even suicide. Research shows that the mere presence of a mobile device can detract from interpersonal interactions by interfering with depth of conversation and closeness.[25]

Identify the people with whom you hold meaningful interpersonal relationships. How are relationships different at home, at work and in other aspects of your daily life? Who are the individuals with whom you interact impersonally? Identify appropriate times for impersonal responses. Impersonal responses allow your life to progress smoothly, but do not maintain or advance interpersonal relationships.

Linkages Between Interpersonal Communication and Health Outcomes

What are the direct ties between interpersonal communication behaviors and health outcomes? A vivid answer is supplied by a study in Sweden in which researchers measured the heart rates of 300 healthy women over a 24-hour period. The women were also surveyed about their network of friends and the extent to which they felt angry or depressed. Heart-rate variability has a wide range among healthy people and has a narrow range in people prone to heart disease. The study found that women who lived alone, with few friends, and with no one to help them in stress-related activities were significantly more likely to have a heart rate with little variation, indicating greater risk of heart problems.[26]

Interpersonal communication has been shown to play an active role in a number of health outcomes including mortality, cardiovascular diseases, cancer and immune system disorders.

Mortality

Researchers keep close track of mortality statistics that reveal the ages at which individuals die and as well as causes of death. The statistics and conclusions resulting from mortality studies provide insights into the relationships between communication and length of life. As Bert N. Uchino concludes after a review of over 200 medical studies:

> Importantly, about 80 percent of the studies I reviewed found an association between . . . (social) support and lower mortality rate. These studies show that individuals low in support appear to have, on average, a two-to-three times greater risk of mortality compared to those high in social support. Thus, the available research provides strong overall evidence that social support is related to lower mortality rate across a variety of diseases.[27]

Cardiovascular Diseases

For years The American Heart Association annually reported around a million heart-related deaths a year; with medical advances, this number has dropped. The association reported on January 21, 2021 that 41 percent of all deaths in 2019 were due to cardiovascular failure. Uchino's review of available research reached the following conclusions:

> 1. Positive relationships with people can be used to predict a lower mortality rate for heart attack victims, even after considering the influence of income, smoking, and disease severity.[28]
>
> 2. Positive relationships are a risk-reducing factor in the development of cardiovascular disease.[29]

Cancer

The second leading cause of death in the U.S., cancer is likely to strike one out of every three of us sometime in our lives. Some forms of cancer are deadlier than others; for example, the five-year survival rate in 2019 for pancreatic cancer was only 4 percent, compared to 85 percent for breast cancer, and 93 percent for prostate cancer.[30] The deadlier forms appear to be influenced less by our social interactions, but other forms are significantly influenced by them. For example, breast cancer patients receiving empathic support from other breast cancer patients in randomly formed support groups, lived about eighteen months longer than those without support. Conversely, well-meaning but anxious family and friends may contribute to greater psychological distress and poorer coping capacities.[31]

Immune System Disorders

Interpersonal relationships have been shown to have both positive and negative influences on the ability of your body to resist infection. On the negative side, interpersonal conflicts are a common cause of stressful environments, including chronic problems at home, at work, and major life events. Laboratory studies have found that experimentally induced marital conflicts suppress cellular components of immune functions, and longitudinal studies have linked family conflict with a higher risk for acquired upper respiratory infections.[32] On the positive side, healthy communication provides many benefits, including facilitating the motivation to provide better care for oneself, provide support, and help regulate emotional responses.[33]

Dr. Jen's Rx

For...

Address...

R_x Date:.........................

Life, just like communication, is not reversible.

Refills NA 1 2 3 4 5

Signature..

Psychologist Sheldon Cohen has confirmed previous studies that suggest that colleagues, relatives, friends, and loved ones can act as a team to protect themselves from the common cold. Cohen found that it is not simply the absolute number of social contacts that is important; equally important are the qualities and nature of the communication. Cohen and his colleagues recruited 151 women and 125 men whom he asked to keep a record of all contacts with people, as well as the nature of their interactions, at least once every two weeks. These voluntary subjects were then exposed to the common cold virus and their rate of infections was recorded. Of those people with fewer and less satisfying interactions , 62 percent developed colds; however, of those subjects who had six or more quality interactions, only 35 percent developed a cold. Cohen theorizes that one of the reasons for the greater immunity is that positive relationships and positive communication induces a "feel good factor" that boosts the ability of the immune system to fight invading viruses.[34] Obviously high-quality interactions involve healthy communication, which includes honesty, mutual trust, empathic listening, and regard for the wellbeing of each other.

Cohen conducted another study to determine the role of happiness and other positive emotions on health. This study confirms that people who are happy, lively, calm, or exhibit other positive emotions, are less likely to become ill when they are exposed to a cold virus than those who report few of these emotions. When they do come down with a cold, happy people report fewer symptoms than the general population. In contrast, the population reporting more negative emotions such as depression, anxiety, and anger was associated with catching colds. That study, however, left open the possibility that the greater resistance to infectious illness among happier people may not have been due to happiness, but rather to other characteristics that are often associated with reporting positive emotions such as optimism, extraversion, feelings of purpose in life and self-esteem.[35]

While there is a need for much more work to be done to validate the linkages between our communication behaviors and our physical health, there seems to be little question that healthy communication can help us live happier, healthier, and longer lives.[36]

Personal Reflections

1. Conduct a self-inventory of your communication behavior.
   a. Are you a good listener? Do you try to perceive the other's feelings and share feedback?
   b. What qualities do you look for in choosing possible friends? Which are most essential?
   c. Are your behaviors congruent? Do you say what you mean and reinforce the message with appropriate nonverbal behaviors?
   d. Are you a good team player? Do you work for cooperation including being willing to compromise?
2. In what ways did your life changes caused by the 2020 pandemic impact your interpersonal communication.
3. How do you employ social media to enhance your interpersonal communication?
4. Do you ever inappropriately treat loved ones, individuals on-line or fellow workers in impersonal ways? Can you identify patterns of behavior that you might like to change?

Chapter 3 - The Evolution of the Human Brain

A three-pound lump of wrinkled tissue with no joints, valves, or moving parts serves as the motherboard of your body's other systems and gives you the capacity to think and, in a very real sense, to exist. It is the center for all the connections and relatedness of all components of your life. Twenty-first century neuroscience has opened the brain to us as never before. While the brain can be sub-divided into zones and functions, the lines of demarcation are blurred. If a person loses vision, the lobe that processes light may repurpose itself for other senses. After a stroke, the area that controls the arms may transfer to another area. Flexibility and adaptability are key capacities of the brain.

The human brain is an exceedingly complex organ that has evolved over millions of years. The earliest and deepest area of the animal brainstem dates back 500 million years when reptiles dominated the world. This "reptilian brain" was primarily concerned with the fundamental biological stability of the organism and managed only the simplest tasks of life support – heart rate, breathing, and reacting to life-threatening dangers such as predators.

About 200 to 300 million years later, some creatures started to undertake a transition from sea-dwelling to living on land, so a new brain started to evolve. The variation of changing environments on land, the demands of gravity, and the issue of finding food and drink prompted the brain to develop a limbic system, a group of cell structures sitting immediately atop the brainstem. This area of the brain regulates such functions as the maintenance of body temperature, hormone balances, heart rate, and blood sugar levels. It is responsible for much more than just controlling recurrent internal processes. In mammals, the limbic system controls the elaborate reactions that have to do with survival, such as choosing to fight or flee in order to preserve life. The limbic system also controls the hypothalamus, the "brain of the brain," which regulates eating, drinking, sleeping, waking, hormone balances, heart rate, body temperature, sex, and, for the first time, emotions. Out of necessity, the hypothalamus operates on "auto pilot" and requires no conscious choices as it fulfills physiological needs.

Through a combination of chemical and electrical messages, the hypothalamus directs the master gland of the brain, the pituitary. This gland regulates the body through hormones, which are chemicals manufactured and secreted by special neurons in the brain and carried through the blood to targets in the body. Internal feedback provides the basis for regulation. If an animal's blood is too cool, the hypothalamus stimulates heat production and conservation.

The next portion of the brain to develop and evolve was the cerebral cortex, thought to have appeared about 50 million years ago. This late brain performs the functions that increase adaptability and execute the capacities that define us as human. In the cortex, decisions are made; the external and internal world is organized; individual experiences are stored in memory; speech is produced and understanding of symbolism is made possible; sounds are heard and replicated in such forms as music; and paintings are created and understood. The cortex is thin and greatly enfolded to fit into the relatively small head of a human. The cortex is responsible for making decisions and judgments on all the information coming from the body as well as from the outside world. As these messages are received, they are compared to existing memories, and the cerebral cortex determines whether a new memory is formed. It then triggers either an unconscious response or conscious consideration. Most human actions can be controlled by the cortex through developed self-regulation. Problems develop when humans persist in using their limbic brain and stay on auto-pilot, rather than override it by making a calculated response from the cerebral cortex.

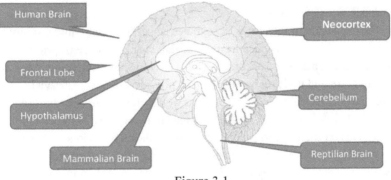

Figure 3.1

The latest step in the evolutionary path is the neocortex ("new bark"), which governs higher cognitive behaviors. It is said to make up 80 percent of the human brain today.[37] These controllable behaviors are reliant upon billions of tiny brain cells called "neurons" that are separated by small gaps called "synapses." These spaces are inhabited by a variety of chemical substances such as dopamine, serotonin, and noradrenalin, which stimulate each neuron to connect with other neurons to control the stream of information. Over the millions of years of evolution, these synaptic transmissions have grown in complexity to meet the needs of our increasingly complex human brains.

Two parts of the brain on which we will focus most of our discussion are the limbic system, which controls emotion and feeling, and the prefrontal cortex, the most forward portion of the brain, which is the thinking part of the brain. The prefrontal cortex is supposed to oversee and help regulate the limbic system, but sometimes we fail to use this capacity and get unintended consequences. Fortunately, research has shown that change is possible in the interactions and communications between these two areas of the brain, and this change leads to more healthy outcomes.[38]

As noted, the billions of tiny nerve cells known as neurons provide the communication and computing power in the brain like tiny microchips. Neurons are constantly talking to each other by firing electrical pulses to create synapses. Neuroscientists are interested in the network of communication neurons called neural circuits that work together like a series of connected computers.[39] Human brain growth occurs as both a natural and a learned activity (both nature and nurture). At a foundational level, the genetic code contained in DNA provides a template for the construction of the uniform structures of the nervous system, while the next level, genetic transcription, allows the brain to be shaped and reshaped by learning acquired through experiences. There's a good chance that the reason the human species is developing a larger and more complex brain is that doing so increases the probability of survival of our species. More complex brain functioning provides a greater variety of responses across diverse environments that, in turn, enhance the probability of survival.

The expansion of the cortex in primates corresponds with increasingly larger social groups. As humans became more social, changes in needs, priorities, brain functioning, and behaviors occurred. A need for cooperation developed and people began to share and trade resources. Parents provide extended supervision of their young and people begin to protect others as well as themselves. The brain expanded in maternal programming and societal connections. A need for understanding one another created the need to predict and judge other's behaviors as friend or foe. Self-awareness, and emotions expanded.[40] Along with self-awareness came the need to discover and convey ourselves, our beliefs, and our emotions.

Humans have evolved and are in the process of evolving. We maintain the basic reptilian inclination for personal survival, but the evolving human brain has also become hardwired with a need to connect with others. There are times when the lower reptilian brain reflexes suspend the more preferred, more evolved reflective responses. The brain is integrative in nature, allowing communication between different parts, prioritizing functions, and allowing a segment to take the lead according to what it perceives as happening at any one given time. The brain is always active. It urges the body to respond to stimuli unconsciously, or it calls for conscious attention to matters of concern, potential threats, and things that are out of the ordinary.

Integration and participation of the different parts of the human brain is essential to existence and continuing evolution. One problem that exists at the present level of brain evolution is that the instinctive high alert system does not necessarily distinguish between the real, remembered, or fantasized stimuli that trigger emotions. Nor does the brain always recognize the differences between physical threats and social threats (such as insults).

Louis Cozintino points out that when overwhelmed by traumatic experiences, brains lose the ability to maintain neural integration across the various networks dedicated to behavior, emotion, sensation, and conscious awareness. Cognitive neuroscientists consider the basal forebrain a kind of default network because when an individual feels threatened, this portion of the brain abandons its other tasks and puts the body on high alert so that we can fight, flee, or freeze. Social neuroscientists refer to this same system as a shared circuit, noting that certain of its neurons fire in the same way regardless of whether an action is completed by oneself or observed being completed by another (some neurobiologists suggest that this could be a neurological empathetic response). It is far too early to tell for certain, but it appears empathy may be a societal survival skill to be added to the arsenal of fighting, running and freezing. At present, however, empathy is not the response of impulse when a person feels threatened.

The human brain, as we have suggested, was originally designed for survival, not for thinking. Humans began to group together, and their brains began to adapt to the complexities of social order. From prenatal days forward, the brain has been programming systems to respond immediately to "danger signs," mostly as reflex and, therefore, without conscious thought. These automatic responses save people from imminent danger, but are capable of leading to regrettable erroneous action –a fight resulting from a perceived insult, or even the shooting of a family member mistaken for an intruder.

As the brain perceives an imminent threat such as encountering a dangerous animal, it guides you to flee (retreat), blend into the background so you won't be noticed (freeze), or go on the defensive (fight.) Those processes worked well for non-social animals, but as social interactions began and continue to be an essential aspect of the human make-up, reflective thought becomes essential. Those attributes considered most human,--language, perception, creativity and intelligence--represent only a small fraction of the evolving brain's functions. If you want to shift from automatic reactions that originate in your limbic brain to more deliberate responses, your brain must be retrained to consciously evaluate its choices and the consequences of those choices.

The Automatic System and the Reflective System

As noted, the two brain processing systems manage an extraordinary amount of information bombarding the senses at any one time. The automatic processing system is a primal system geared toward detecting danger, prompting immediate action, keeping you safe from immediate harm, and ignoring sensations it deems "inconsequential." The deliberate reflective processing system allows for more time-consuming reflection. It allows you, in safety, to consider the appropriateness of your responses.

The **automatic response system** is "on" all the time, taking in as many sensations as it can: sifting, sorting, dismissing, responding and forwarding information to the deliberate reflective processing system for delayed but more complex considerations and responses. This is a primitive "short cut" to quickly assess information and detect dangerous situations in need of quick response.

When sensations do not fall into existing schemas and interpretations/responses cannot be instantly accessed, instinct errs on the side of caution, and a defensive stance is automatically taken. The default automatic reaction to confusion or to unfamiliar experience is defensiveness. The automatic system is useful as an immediate alert, allowing us to get out of harm's way or to defend ourselves, but it does not allow in-depth analysis of a situation.

If you see a car moving toward you, you may not think, "There is a car driving toward me. I must take evasive action." Instead, your eyes and ears sense the car and your *automatic survival response* moves you to get out of harm's way. You may not even remember moving your body, just seeing the car. The message was simple: "Danger, flee!" Repeated interpretations and emotional responses are also created by forging neural pathways. If your sister has a history of telling you, in a particular tone of voice, that she wants to talk to you and you tend to associate that tone of voice and phrase with being degraded and bossed around (and the thought of that makes you angry), you may start to skip the progressive thoughts and jump straight from her "Let's talk," to becoming angry. These triggers and immediate emotional responses can cause problems as the circumstances or the people with whom you interact change. Responses often replicate obsolete judgments and utilize interpretations of which you are no longer conscious. Protective rapid response is the primary goal of the expedited response system.

One example of improperly trained judgments is in the use of stereotypes. Stereotyping occurs when judgments are made and people are categorized without allowing those generalizations to be revised. It is natural to categorize information and what you know about people as you make inferences regarding them. Stereotyping takes this inclination too far. For example, during the 2020 pandemic, Asians were subjected to discriminatory behavior including racist slurs and hostile behavior.

Compared to the automatic response system, the reflective response system is slower. It considers multiple complex interpretations before selecting one response to what you see, hear, smell, taste and feel. Reflective responses are processed consciously. It is possible to override automatic responses by retraining the brain with reflective responses and employing them repeatedly until the brain becomes reprogrammed. Such responses are a central agent for individual empowerment. Through reflection, you assume responsibility and power over your emotions. Whereas automatic interpreting occurs constantly, individuals *decide* to respond reflectively, so their reactions are dependent on conscious thought. During the reflective process, individuals consider each step in the perception process, accepting or rejecting conclusions of the original thinking process and determining where deeper consideration is needed. Automatic and reflective processes are compared in Table 3.1.

Neurologists report that there are methods to "retrain" your responses. You can distinguish more carefully those things presently perceived as dangers. All threats are typically lumped together. If, however, you teach your protective system that a particular phenomenon, like being criticized, poses no immediate danger, and will, in fact, help you, in this case, become better at your job, you may be able to stifle the immediate desire to defend yourself. Another strategy is to interrupt unhelpful habitual short cuts and replace them with new consciously constructed deliberative reflections until those new responses become habits. You can remove or avoid "triggers." This is why "weekends away" can be beneficial to marriages and long-term relationships. Partners in new environments have removed themselves from many of their emotional triggers and have a better chance to forge healthy interactions that they may use to supersede old triggers and negative responses. The most recent research suggests that you can change even the most deeply rooted habitual responses (of say, obsessive-compulsive disorders) when you introduce a goal held in higher esteem than the old habit. Visualizing the goal helps to break habits. So, just as the person who moves to a new home in the same town, tired and lost in thought at the end of a work day, may, out of habit, head for their former residence, that person can replace that habit with the goal of arriving at their new residence, rather than the old habit of automatically navigating "home."[41]

Since you are able to retrain your brain in beneficial ways, it is your responsibility to determine what retraining will help you the most. Police training now includes retraining of the brain for recruits to more quickly size up circumstances and pertinent aspects of a situation such as distinguishing items in a hand (is it a phone or a gun?), as an override for a societal tendency to shoot based on stereotypes taught by our culture.

| TABLE 3.1 - AUTOMATIC AND REFLECTIVE PROCESSING ||
AUTOMATIC	REFLECTIVE
Unconscious judgmental system for removing the body from imminent dangerous situations.	Conscious reflective system for considering and determining actions when faced with new or confusing situations.
Judges, interprets, prompts responses.	Ponders, evaluates, reevaluates, refines responses and retrains automatic responses.
Fast, immediate responses.	Slower processing.
Handles huge quantities of sensations quickly (almost instantaneously).	Processes many sensations but fewer and more slowly than automatic responses.
Alerts the reflective system of sensations that require greater consideration but puts system on high alert until phenomenon is determined to be safe.	Takes over the processing of sensations that cannot be referenced easily by the automatic system.
Continually occurring.	Occurs by choice.
Determines initial reactions and drives unconscious responses. Overrides reflective system when preserving self.	Can consciously override automatic responses by *retraining* the brain.
Recognizes repeated responses and forms habits and shortcuts	Can short-circuit habits by injecting goals.
Shortcuts from sensation to judgment, emotional/physical response and/or action.	Proceeds through a series of steps: attend, organize, interpret, respond emotionally, respond physically (action).
Frequently occurs at the unconscious level.	Consists of conscious deliberation.
Simplifies decisions by utilizing binary decisions and judgments (black/white, dangerous/safe, respond/don't respond).	Capable of assuming multiple perspectives and considering complex aspects of situations (perceived "gray" areas).
Responds with one of four responses: 1) safe/step down, 2) danger/fight, 3) danger/flee, 4) danger, freeze or hide.	Capable of creating decisions for appropriate actions and considering alternatives.
Overrides other systems when threats are perceived.	Does not function well when brain is in high alert.
Tied to extreme emotions, actions and loss of control.	Allows individuals to rule their emotions rather, than emotions ruling them.

The most significant aspect of *conscious reflection* is that it is the center of empowerment for individuals in their communicating. Through the reflective process, you can give up unhealthy automatic interpretations and unhealthy responses. Rather than "Shoot first, ask questions later," you can question the reasons for emotional responses and, by instituting new, more accurate, healthier interpretations, respond in ways that promote healthier decisions, relationships, and actions.

Interacting with another individual is more than a simple act of progressing through a series of mental tasks. In both individuals, the body and mind work as a team. The body receives and sends messages, and the mind sorts, interprets, and forms responses. These are not discreet processes. Recently, researchers have discovered that while individuals are engaged in interpersonal activity with each other, their neural activity responds to each other in a kind of "dance" that, when practiced, forges habitual neural pathways affecting physical, emotional, and relational health.

Processing for Maximum Benefit

Repeated or extremely noteworthy experiences, whether responded to automatically or reflectively, establish neural patterns or habitual responses on which future automatic responses are made. Repeating responses adds reinforcement. Have you ever noticed yourself responding automatically to situations and not knowing why you acted or felt as you did? Sometimes those responses benefited you; at other times, they interfered with positive actions or interactions with others. But you can identify sensory "triggers" for emotional and physical behaviors, and use conscious reflective processing to "reprogram" more appropriate automatic responses.

You can reinforce effective automatic responses, such as including alternative interpretations and reprogramming ineffectual automatic responses or overriding inappropriate responses with more reasonable ones. For example, in women's self-defense classes, women are encouraged to notice circumstances and surroundings to avoid unnecessarily dangerous situations (situations that may have been judged as "safe" because they had never been attacked in them before). Women are encouraged to immediately key into automatic feelings of danger or discomfort, and to replace existing programmed habitual behaviors of decorum with less "ladylike" behaviors. These women reprogram immediate physical responses to specific dangerous situations in ways that would not be acceptable in other circumstances. In order to become proficient, they practice until these responses "come naturally." This change accomplished through deliberately identifying appropriate specific sensory cues and appropriate responses, and then practicing responses until neural patterns forge a short cut from sensory input to behavioral response that is acceptable only in this vulnerable situation.

Along with psychologists, you can learn to understand the importance of self-regulation, and grow to control your own welfare, or the welfare of individuals with whom interact. Conscious reflection allows you to realize that your initial interpretations of situations may be limited, and that factors not under your control may influence another person's response to you. While you can't assume responsibility for another individual's action, interpretations, or responses, you can most certainly assume responsibility for your own.

Self-regulation

Everyone occasionally responds inappropriately to sensory stimuli. You might, for example, carelessly respond to someone and unintentionally upset that individual. You might accept another's words or actions as a devaluing of your own self-worth. You might choose an immediate gratification over a delayed greater reward, (for example, going into debt to purchase something now rather than waiting until you have earned the money or until the item is sold for a price within your budget). At other times, you may respond in a way that you know is not in your own interest. Everyone does this sometimes; "eating this cookie will delay the weight loss I've been striving for, but I'm going to have it anyway." Everyone occasionally responds in regrettable ways because of poor judgment, reflexive response, or just plain not knowing better.

People are so used to touching their faces (an easy way of spreading germs from hands to mouth, nose and eyes) that they had to be retrained to stop this habit during the 2020 pandemic. Social distancing also forced modifications of touching and moving close to others.

Habitual or repeated inability to recognize or resist urges that get you into trouble, harm you, or harm others is unhealthy. When impulsive actions interfere with your life, they are considered pathological. This includes many conditions, such as ADHD, obsessive-compulsive disorders, antisocial personality disorder, borderline personality disorder, addictions, eating disorders, pathological over-spending, pathological under-spending, intermittent explosive disorder, kleptomania, pyromania, pathological gambling, sexual addiction, or self-inflicted bodily damage such as cutting oneself, pulling one's own hair out, and compulsive scab picking.

Self-regulation, self-restraint, self-discipline, self-control, or impulse control are all terms that refer to the processes used to manage drives and emotions. Appropriate self-regulation is important for a variety of reasons.

The aspect of self-regulation known as **ego control** is instrumental in building and maintaining meaningful relationships. It is an essential component in empathizing as you set aside your own perspectives long enough to take on the perspectives of another. You can monitor the coding of messages sent by matching another individual's "code book" so a message will be interpreted as intended.

Self-regulation promotes emotional well-being by fostering **ego resiliency,** the ability to recover from inevitable blows to your ego. Sometimes people need a strong enough self-concept to recover from intentional attacks made by someone else, but often an insult or criticism is perceived where none was intended. Either way, self-disciplined communicators develop the ability to consciously examine their own emotional responses to people, circumstances, and events. In this way, an individual identifies "triggering events" that bring about habitual emotional and physical responses. This further enables that individual to question the validity of unidentified interpretations on which the emotional and physical responses are based. Individuals can even institute plans for changing communication behaviors that interfere with achieving personal life goals by intentionally shifting unhelpful automatic responses to conscious reflective responses.

Self-regulation in the form of **intellectual discipline** develops and maintains intellectual ability. Students who are not disciplined enough to study can find themselves dropping out of college. Employees who don't show up to work can find themselves unemployed. Critical thinking is disciplining oneself to reasonably and logically question what one is told before accepting it as truth. Researchers have discovered that older individuals who regularly exercise their brain with intellectual exercises such as puzzles (word search, logic puzzles, crossword puzzles), games (bridge or poker), by regularly learning new things (a language or skill), or by practicing creative problem-solving are less likely to suffer from dementia. Likewise, physical fitness, through regulation of exercise and appetite, promotes both good health and a sense of emotional well-being. Neither too much nor too little is healthy.

Self-regulation is essential to cooperatively create outcomes greater than might be reachable alone. You must at times override your own impulses and interpretations to create something greater than you are able to by yourself. Consider societies and their achievements from ancient marvels such as the pyramids to contemporary achievements such as the number of people helped by "Comic Relief." On the job, you regulate your contributions to meet the needs of your employer. You discipline yourself to show up when you are expected, to meet deadlines, to behave in ways deemed "appropriate," and to interact with others so you can effectively work together. Very few people work alone in a vacuum, so it is crucial to develop self-discipline. A lack of self-regulation can be blamed for many societal outrages such as bullying, cheating, road rage, and even school shootings,

According to extensive research, while we typically underestimate babies' ability to understand and communicate before they begin speaking, we tend to overestimate the brain power of walking, talking toddlers.[42] As early as six months of age, a child can be affected by a parent's depression or anxiety and by marital squabbles. By about ten months, babies start to add meaning to the language they're used to hearing. Parents are encouraged to use real words in grammatically complete sentences, not "baby talk."[43]

Many parents believe their child should learn to share at age two, but this skill doesn't typically develop until age three or four. This step is part of what is known as "theory of mind." Theory of mind is the ability to differentiate one's own perspective and preferences from those of someone else. The classic experiment in theory of mind is known as the "Sally-Ann" test. A child is told that Sally has a basket and Ann has a box. Sally puts an apple in her basket, and then leaves the room. Ann moves the apple to the box. The child is then asked where Sally will look for the apple when she returns. Correctly answering that Sally will look in her basket shows that the child understands that he/she has a different perspective than Sally. This capacity is important for developing empathy, making friends, and doing well academically.[44]

According to a group of cognitive psychologists in a 2015 report, most parents believe that two-year-old children can control their emotions and impulses. Yet children have very limited self-control until they are four. When toddlers won't stop throwing tantrums, doing something forbidden, or refusing to share, they aren't being obstinate but rather haven't yet developed the capacity for self-control. Strategies such as distracting the child with a favorite toy while passing candy in the grocery store checkout line can help with issues of self-control. In dealing with a tantrum, attempt to identify and acknowledge the child's feelings by putting them into words. Tantrums are sometimes triggered by feelings of not being understood. Empathy can assist in identifying causation.[45]

Rigorous scientific testing indicates that self-regulation is like a muscle. It can be consciously exercised and strengthened.[46] Children who are taught how to regulate their behaviors, whether in school or from their parents, experience greater success in school, in relationships, and as adults. Children benefit most from parents who teach through patient discussion and consistent example.[47] Attempts to teach self-regulation by punishing children who are "at risk" (have genetic predispositions to have problems with self-regulation) are not successful. In fact, punishment actually seems to make it more difficult for these children to self-regulate. The earlier the training begins and the more training a child receives, the greater the positive influence on their lives as young adults.[48]

Recall that impulse control is managed by the prefrontal lobe, the area of the brain that enables conscious reflective thought. The frontal lobe and amygdala control inhibition and judgment and recognize possible consequences related to immediate actions. These specialized parts of the brain develop during childhood and adolescence, but they are not fully wired until about the age of twenty. Connections in your brain develop from the back to the front, and those important for higher-order thinking continue to form and strengthen into a person's twenties. During the teen years, the midbrain, important for emotion, sexual functioning, learning and memory, is hyperactive. As teens transition into adulthood, connections in the front of their brain are strengthened while those in the other regions are reduced in potency A fully developed frontal lobe is essential for planning, decision making, impulse control and risk avoidance.[49] These parts of the brain may be strengthened with practice throughout adulthood or weakened by head injury, psychiatric illness and substance abuse, (particularly alcohol), as well as other factors.

Self-Control can be worn out.[50] Perhaps this is the reason stress, caffeine, alcohol and traumatic experiences contribute to impulsive behaviors. We do know that after being depleted, self-control can then be replenished. However, the actual physiological process of replenishing self-control has not been identified completely. There is research to suggest that sleep and positive emotional experiences such as humor, laughter, affirmation and warm experiences with others can help to restore self-control. Scientists have long searched in vain for a class of brain cells that can explain the linkage of sensory perception and memory that provides immediate recognition when we see a familiar face. Neuroscientists at Rockefeller University in 2021 have identified a collection of cells in the brain's temporal pole that specializes in familiar face recognition. This discovery will likely help us to devise strategies to help people to improve their abilities of face recognition.

Multiple Intelligences

Howard Gardner introduced the idea of MULTIPLE INTELLIGENCES, now generally accepted by sociologists, psychologists and educators. There are six primary intelligences: **Abstract Intelligence** is the kind of intellect that is measured on IQ tests. **Social Intelligence** involves understanding people and interacting well with them. It leads to successful relationships. **Practical Intelligence** encompasses the ability to do what needs to be done and is frequently referred to as "common sense." **Emotional Intelligence** includes "self-awareness and the management of the inner experience." **Aesthetic Intelligence** is the holistic ability to respond to artistic aspects of life (such as appreciating line and form in architecture, texture, flow, and color of clothing, or the beauty of the human form) and art forms (including visual arts, literature, dance, music, theatre).[51] **Kinesthetic Intelligence** coordinates the entire body in experiences such as athletic endeavors, playing musical instruments, dancing, or driving a car.[52]

Kinds of Intelligence

- Abstract Intelligence
- Aesthetic Intelligence
- Kinesthetic Intelligence
- Emotional Intelligence
- Social Intelligence
- Practical Intelligence

Ideally, an individual has high intelligence in six and is able to draw on them individually and collectively as needed; but everyone has strengths and weaknesses. You develop and expand your competencies in all areas, and you nurture your abilities to integrate intelligences. Identify the intelligence types that are your strengths and the ones in which you feel weakest.

In 1994, Dr. Daniel Goleman made a significant contribution to our understanding and acceptance of multiple intelligence with the publication of his book *Emotional Intelligence (Why It Can Matter More Than I.Q.)* In it he identifies a crucial set of human capacities that allow us to manage our emotions and enhance our potential for positive relationships.[53] We recommend it to you for this important insight.

Goleman followed his 1994 publication with *Social Intelligence* in 2006 in which he synthesizes the findings of neuroscience that suggest humans are "wired to connect" with other people. He suggests interpersonal relations have a biological impact on the body, releasing hormones that affect immune systems, hearts, and brains. Good relationships are like vitamins, and bad relationships are like poison. You may be as susceptible to other people's emotions as you are to their colds. Isolation or relentless stress can be life-shortening. Fortunately, Goleman believes humans have a built-in bias toward empathy, cooperation, and altruism if you appropriately nurture and develop your social intelligence.[54]

Communication, like your health, centers on interpretations and decisions, both conscious and unconscious. The empowered communicator balances automatic and reflective thinking processes in all six areas of intelligence.

Personal Reflections

1. Identify the kinds of intelligences that are your strengths and weaknesses. Can you think of ways you can use this knowledge in your daily life?

2. How did self-regulation manifest itself for you during the 2020 pandemic?

3. Assumptions are beliefs that you take for granted. They usually operate at a subconscious level. Consider more deeply the assumptions you make in daily life:

   A. What do you take for granted?
   B. What is being assumed in a news story?
   C. What are assumptions you make about close friends, parents, children?
   D. Do you tend to ascribe good motives to others or are you suspicious?
   E. Are you assuming some things you shouldn't?
   F. Consider arguments that seem logical but you disagree with their conclusions. Are there assumptions you do not fully accept?

34

SECTION II – FIRST KEY: AUTHENTICITY

Chapter 4 - Determining Reality, Right and Wrong

The capacity to experience the world gives life its personal meaning. When you experience fully (in keeping with the theme of this book, we could say "healthfully") and respond authentically to those experiences, your life is exceedingly rich. Other individuals are an essential aspect of your existence, and experiencing of others occurs only through communication. Healthy interpersonal communication is dependent upon your ability to embrace and respond to each unique communication moment spontaneously and wisely, a process which, in turn, requires consciousness of self, other persons and the world. Such consciousness is developed in an ongoing process throughout one's lifetime.

Human Consciousness

Consciousness refers to your capacity not only to perceive, remember, think about and imagine the world, but also to distinguish between and reflect upon values you place on the experience. It is possible to distinguish between memories and present experiences. Consciousness is related to your welfare. The individual walking alone at night lost in thought is in more danger of being attacked than the individual consciously aware of surroundings. A loss of capacity to discriminate between different levels of awareness is frequently associated with confusion and psychological difficulties associated with mental health.

Philosophers have long studied human consciousness from a perspective of intentionality in the human experience. This term does not refer to such matters as the intention to go to the theatre or to read a book. Instead, it refers to the assertion that human consciousness is always aware of something. *Consciousness is continuous and ongoing.* If you are not conscious of anything, then you are unconscious. If you are conscious, you are aware of something and this something has meaning. You name it, think about it, remember it, imagine some of its possibilities, and have feelings about it.

An experience is always of some content, such as a person's face, or the sound of a voice, or the recollections of someone's actions, that has meaning to you. Another basic characteristic of experience is that, whether occurring in the present or as a memory, experience always has an emotional quality. Thus, my memory of my father is accompanied by feelings of warmth, nostalgia, and good humor as I recall some of our conversations. A flirtatious look from an individual I find attractive is accompanied by aesthetic and sensual feelings.

So, the conscious communicator is aware of the following influences on perception: 1) the influence of past on present experiences, 2) the distinction between a lived experience and a memory, 3) reasons exist for all responses (whether those reasons are valid or not is another issue), and 4) both content and emotional reaction are a part of experiencing. Understanding these influences lead the conscious communicator to an important conclusion: individuals may share an activity yet have completely different experiences. Your particular point of view or perception of a single conscious experience is a combination of many factors that fuse with the present circumstances.

What is the difference between conscious and unconscious thoughts? Some kinds of information in your brain are conscious, such as what you are now seeing and hearing, your plans for the day, and some messages you are sending to others. You ponder conscious thoughts, discuss them, and let them guide your behaviors in a deliberate manner. But the brain also guides unconscious behavior – our heart rate, the muscle control that lets us walk and hold a pencil, and the nonverbal signals that accompany messages we generate; these tend to be sealed off from our planning and reasoning circuits, operating as reflexes.

One of the recent discoveries of neuroscientists is the idea that all our thoughts, sensations, joys and pleasures, aches and pains consist entirely of physiological activities that are located in the tissue of the brain.[55] With functional MRI, cognitive neuroscientists can interpret a person's thoughts by observing the blood flow in his/her brain. They can determine the content of a picture the person is looking at, or if the person is thinking about a particular place. Physical manipulation of the brain can also impact consciousness. Electrical stimulations of the brain during surgery can cause a person to hallucinate or have memories such as learning a song or reliving a childhood birthday party. We also know how certain chemicals affect the brain; from caffeine to alcohol, to drugs such as LSD – they alter how a person thinks, sees and feels.

Why are certain aspects of your consciousness accessible and deliberative, while others are hidden and automatic? To keep you safe and to avoid information overload, the brain has developed a system of expedited processing. The brain's main function is to keep your body functioning. To do that, the brain monitors and maintains all bodily functions as well as maintaining constant surveillance of all that surrounds you. The brain sorts sensations, delegating them to the parts of the brain best suited to processing and responding.

Just as you can be overwhelmed by many people making demands of you at the same time, the decision circuits inside your brain would be swamped if every movement and action you take had to be determined deliberately. Recall how many things you had to *think* about as you were learning to drive an automobile. Now that you've been driving for a while many of your movements are completed automatically. The key to the brain's processing is to maintain focus and be able to differentiate between matters that should receive automatic response, and those that should be considered in a deliberate, reflective way.

The Attribution of Reality to Our Experiences

One of the fundamental distinctions we make regarding experience is distinguishing between reality and unreality. Every society is based on a set of assumptions about what is real. Reality is usually assumed to be what can be perceived and validated, and tends to be associated with the physical world. Reality is what an individual or group identify as fact. In the one woman show, *The Search for Intelligent Life in the Universe,* Lily Tomlin's humorously philosophical bag lady proclaims that reality is nothing but "a collective hunch." Reality is associated with truth and fact. Facts are verifiable. Truth consists of the reporting of fact. The ability to distinguish between reality and fantasy is associated with mental health. The habit of telling the truth is associated with honesty. The ability to incorporate facts with sound reasoning leads to critical thinking and sound conclusions. Acknowledging a phenomenal reality is crucial for sanity and judgments concerning fairness, justice and personal conduct.

Reality is an attribution that is an act or judgment formed by a person, imbuing the experience with the quality of reality that must be reckoned with. By the same token, we can withdraw our attribution of reality from another experience and view it as not real. Thus, I may waken from a deep sleep with a conviction that someone is trying to harm me. Upon awakening, however, I reflect upon this experience and say with relief, "It was not real. It was only a dream. No one is really trying to harm me." In much the same way, I may experience myself as being trapped by a domineering parent until I perceive my own power in the situation and "see" the situation differently.

No two people experience the world in the same way. It follows that if there are four billion human beings in the world, there are four billion ways in which the world is experienced. If each person embodies a unique perspective, then it is a momentous thing to validate perspectives of reality. Changes in the world regarding human rights, whether the topic is African exploitation, treatment of Native Americans, or the limited rights imposed upon women in our culture, have been based upon changing perspectives of values, morality, ethics and reality. Conversations between people may raise the question of whose perspective will prevail. Views of what is real, what is important and what is possible are exchanged. Individual perspectives of reality are influenced and altered as we communicate with others.[56]

Perceiving the World

The act of assigning meaning to our sensations is referred to as **perception**. Communication scholars and psychologists tell us that the perceptual process involves six actions: (1) sensing, (2) acknowledging certain signals as significant while discounting others, (3) organizing the sensory input into meaningful groups, (4) decoding by assigning meaning to the sensory input, (5) responding to interpretations emotionally, and (6) responding to interpretations physically.

Here's an example of how this might work: As you sit in a conference room during the first cold day of autumn, a number of sensations bombard you, among which are the pleasant odor of the shampoo used by the young woman sitting next to you, the sound of a maintenance worker raking the grounds beneath the window, the feel of your chair beneath you, the remainder of the mint you popped into your mouth, and the person on the other side of you who you see fidgeting in your peripheral vision. As sensations accost you, you unconsciously note them, dismiss them as insignificant, and focus instead on your notes and your team leader's words, voice, and actions. As you write notes in your notebook, you smell an odor that does not belong here. You become aware of the odor and try to figure out what it means.

This is a significant sensation worthy of attention and reaction. You identify a specific burning smell that you have sensed before. This smell could mean any number of things and warrants different actions according to its ultimate meaning. Could the smell indicate a fire in the building? Should you call the boss's attention to the smell? Evacuate the room? Notify the fire department? As you access your past experiences to interpret the smell, you access schemas or categories of smells. This is a "burning smell," but you are unsure of what specific kind, so you compare it to fires you know: burning food, kitchen fire, burning leaves, bonfire, overheating curling iron, electrical wiring. When have you smelled that smell before? Then understanding strikes! You've smelled this before when the furnace is turned on, after being off for a long time. The accumulated dust is burning off. That's what you interpret this sensation to mean.

The initial anxiety over smelling smoke is calmed, and you decide that your best course of action is to sit back and concentrate on the leader again rather than comment to anyone else or interrupt the meeting. Although you still smell the odor, you attempt to forget or discount it as you once more concentrate on the meeting.

SENSING—Your sense organs, like a television with many channels, permit you to receive a multi-faceted view of the world. With your eyes, you receive the **visual** impressions of objects that are transmitted by light reflection. The human eye scans millions of bits of data per second. Your ears receive the **aural** sense of sound: sensations brought about by vibration. Your nose introduces the **olfactory** sense of smell and, in combination with your **gustatory** sense of taste, you sense aromas and flavors emitted by things. Your touch receptors provide a **tactile** sense for receiving impressions produced by direct physical contact, texture, pressure and pain. You have **thermal** receptors in your skin to detect temperature.

The state of your muscles and joints and the location of your hands, arms, legs and feet are **kinetically** sensed and communicated automatically to your internal sense organs to such a degree that you respond physically to thoughts and memories. Your **kinesthetic** sense provides the ability to feel yourself in motion. Your position in relation to vertical posture is mediated by receptors located in the canals of your ears. Also, the condition of your body's comfort and discomfort, including your need to eat, is detected and received throughout the organs of your body. Your experiences begin with the sensations received from the world around you.

Individuals differ regarding which senses they rely on most for perceiving the world; and physical differences or limitations also individualize your sensory reception. Simply living in different bodies, your sensory reception is different. When we speak of the act of sensing, we are limiting the discussion to the simple act of sensation reaching receptors – sights, smells, sounds, tastes, physical contacts.

ATTENDING—You are bombarded with so many sensations at any one point that it would be impossible to pay attention to all of them at once, so you engage in a filtering activity to determine which sensations are worthy of your attention. Psychologists have spent a great deal of time investigating the various steps involved in perception. They have discovered that you are most likely to attend to sensations associated with danger, movement, or sensations that contrast greatly with other sensations surrounding them (unusual or out-of-place sensations). You also notice sensations that have recently occupied your thoughts.

Your processing system takes in as much as it can from your senses, and it shifts, sorts, files, and sends relevant messages to your conscious reflective processing system. When you are exposed to someone whose appearance or behavior is not consistent with other messages you are receiving, you might find yourself responding without being aware of why: "something about that individual just seems wrong" or "I just couldn't bring myself to trust him" or "I was never comfortable around that person."

DECODING—When you pay attention to the things you sense, you have identified the sensations as significant, and are obliged to endow your sensations with meaning. This process of assigning meaning is known as "decoding," and it requires the actions of *organizing sensations* into meaningful units and *interpreting* those units.

RESPONDING—Just as we have our own unique "dictionary of meanings" reliant upon our past experiences, we also have an entire set of emotional associations linked to our interpretations of experiences, you name the objects and persons in the world and make inferences about what the world is promising (or threatening) to do to you. You experience the world inviting you to do some things and not others, and to behave in certain manners. You *respond emotionally* to those interpretations. Emotions are usually based on a conscious or unconscious interpretation, and are related to your physical response.

Physical responses are exactly that. Your body reacts in response to sensations perceived, interpreted and emotionally responded to. Associated with physical response are nonverbal responses and kinesthetic responses (such as tension in the muscles, changes in blood pressure, and butterflies in the stomach).

You frequently perceive what you expect to perceive. Those who expect to see bad in the world will perceive more negative things than those who expect to see good in the world. Predictive perceptions can actually influence outcomes. Self-fulfilling prophecies are expectations of yourself or others that influence the outcome of an individual's behavior. The individual who believes he/she will succeed will discount a failure as a temporary setback and keep trying until they succeed, while the individual who expects failure is less likely to invest as much energy in trying and is more likely to give up when facing obstacles. Another's expectations also influence outcomes. In a well-known research study, teachers of elementary students were given bogus intelligence scores for students and, by the end of the course, students were matching the teacher's expectations regardless of the students' actual intelligence scores.[57]

What is truly real, and how do we know it? This question has confronted philosophers for thousands of years. The Greek philosopher Plato tried to explain human kind's difficulty with perceiving reality with the allegory about prisoners chained in a cave with no knowledge of the outside world. Plato's prisoners saw reality as the shadows on the wall. There are numerous limitations on our capacity to accurately see and understand our world. Your perceptions are based on your previous experience, language understanding, your current feelings and needs, and the sources of your information. Healthy communication is difficult without similar perceptions of the world and beliefs about it.

Dr. Jen's Rx

For..

Address..

R℞   Date:.......................

There is one mentally ill person who cannot be cured – the one who believes him/herself to be totally healthy.

Refills NA 1 2 3 4 5

Signature..

The nature of language itself, while adding immeasurably to our understanding of the world, paradoxically inhibits our quest for truth. It is sometimes assumed that words, rather than being merely labels, are somehow linked to what they represent. A characteristic of our language permits words to represent things that are ambiguous, abstract, and even misleading.

So called "Reality" television shows are not reality. They tend to be loosely scripted with predictable outcomes. The term "fake news" suggests that you can't believe what you read, confusing reality and fiction. The term originally referred to the practice of creating a fictional text as if it were a real news story. As tabloids such as the National Enquirer have done for years, fictional accounts are presented as actual events. The result is a confusion of reality for uncritical readers and a tendency to discredit fact-based journalism as such.[58]

Your view of the world is often filtered by the source of your "facts." One survey suggests that forty-four percent of Americans get their news from one single source: Facebook! As yet unregulated, Facebook subsidiaries *Newsfeed* and *Trending Topics* are notorious for fictions circulated as factual. It was also discovered that hyper-partisan stories carried on Fox News and Breitbart in 2016 helped disseminate misinformation from Russian cyber-bots.[59]

"Reality testing" means applying the rules of logic and scientific inquiry to everyday life. When you engage in reality testing, you are systematically questioning your initial perceptions or the reports of others until you have scrutinized them more carefully and checked them against evidence.

The pandemic of 2020 provided a memorable example of alternate realities. Then President of the United States, Donald Trump established a daily press briefing that competed with the evening network news time slot. Often there were disagreements in this briefing between the President and his medical advisors. In early briefings, the President was extraordinarily optimistic that the U.S. would see few virus cases and the problem would be short-lived. This was touted even as cases escalated, death tolls mounted and while the expert physicians were telling a different story often at the same briefing. In addition, the President suggested cures such as hydroxychloroquine. While the President repeatedly advised people to try this drug, his medical advisors advised against it due to the lack of significant testing and because of its known cardiac side effects.

In many of the national briefings the President and his advisors expressed different opinions on aspects of the growth and handling of the virus. Many citizens were more confused than illuminated by the daily presentations. The public had to do their own reality testing about the often-opposing ideas, and uncertainty was rampant.

People are by nature uncomfortable admitting they don't know something and lack enough information to make an informed decision. Conversely, it is often scientists and experts that admit uncertainty if the data is not yet available.

Before believing or sharing information of social media, ask yourself such questions as the following: Do I have the hard evidence to know it's true? Does it come from reliable sources? Is the information helpful or useful?" Be careful what you believe to be true because, as long as you believe it, for you it is true.

Looking back to Plato's perspective on the prisoners in a cave, Steven Pinker has suggested optimism as we "catch glimpses of the sunlit world of reality. Even with our infirmities, we have managed to achieve the freedom of a liberal democracy, the wealth of a technological economy, and the truths of modern science."[60] Healthy communication provides the clearest window.

Dr. Hans Rosling, a medical doctor, professor of international health, and a world-renowned advisor to the World Health Organization and UNICEF, administered a test to 12,000 educated adults in 14 countries in 2017. His Book, *Factfulness*,[61] was completed by family in 2018, following his death. The book reveals wide-spread ignorance of basic facts even among the world's highest educated people. Rosling identifies ten instincts that distort our perceptions into thinking that things are worse than they actually are. The thirteen questions that he used for the test were not complicated and contained no trick questions. They focused on the world and how to understand it. Test yourself on this Rosling question: "In the last 20 years, the proportion of the world's population living in extreme poverty has…A. almost doubled, B. remained more or less the same, C. almost halved."

In reality, the proportion of the world's population living in poverty has halved. This basic fact is not known by the majority of the people on earth. On average, only 7 percent of the people who took the test answered correctly. A group of chimpanzees would have guessed the correct answer randomly 33 percent of the time.

Rosling cites ten human instincts that distort our perspective toward the world, like an instinct toward negativity, toward fear, and such tendences as dividing all issues as "us versus them." He offers clear, actionable advice for how to overcome our innate biases and see the world "more factually."

Self-Awareness

The brain of humans evolved to the point of self-awareness, allowing them to recognize their own emotions and values. This unique ability allowed humans to develop the ability to plan strategically based upon their needs, motives and goals toward an anticipated outcome. Healthy behaviors demand that individuals be realistic, neither naively hopeful, nor overly self-critical.

The neural systems responsible for intellect and for emotions are separate yet closely interwoven. Thoughts and feelings are connected, but because of the brain's evolution, the limbic brain (the site of emotions); takes precedence when an individual feels threatened. Fortunately, as discussed in Chapter 3, the prefrontal area has developed the capacity to veto an immediate limbic impulse as it receives and analyzes all parts of the brain. The self-aware person learns to control these emotions: to delay action until all parts of the brain (memory, data, and reason, along with emotions) can contribute to the decision making. Self-awareness can thus work hand-in-hand with self-regulation.

Self-awareness is greatly influenced by other people, starting typically with the parents. The child's beliefs about him/herself are largely derived by listening to what other people say about her/him. Most children are concerned about being seen in a positive light, both in their own eyes and in the eyes of others.

The maintenance of self-esteem is important and the primary tool for maintaining self-esteem is the approval of significant others. Most individuals tend to behave in ways that produce approval and avoid behaving in ways that bring disapproval. Many times, we are tempted to act in ways that will win approval, but are not true to our own inner-feelings or beliefs. One young woman described her behavior as follows:

> I somehow developed a sort of knack, I guess, of well-a-habit-of trying to make people feel at ease around me or to make things go along smoothly.... At a small meeting, I could help things go along nicely and appear to be having a good time. And, sometimes I'd surprise myself by arguing against what I really thought when I saw that the person in charge would be quite unhappy about it if I didn't. I just didn't stand up for my own convictions until I don't know whether I have any convictions to stand up for. I haven't really honestly been being myself, or actually knowing what my real self is, and I've been just playing sort of a false role.[62]

When you perceive that there are parts of yourself eliciting disapproval, you may attempt to hide those parts – if you think it can be done. You then relate to others as "part-persons" rather than whole persons. For example, you may attempt to show no fear except when you are alone. Generally, such attempts are ineffective; people usually see nonverbal signs of tension that are beyond your control, and these are communicated to persons close to you despite your efforts to "say nothing." However, if you are successful in hiding part of yourself, there are two important consequences. The first is that your anger or fear is stored up inside you. You might be able to contain these feelings for a short while but, chances are, they will influence behaviors, confusing both yourself and others when you react to other matters with emotions or actions that seem unrelated. As suppressed emotions accumulate, they erupt in ways that confuse you and your communication partners. Such "breakouts" (or "outbreaks") may not be perceived by you but are easily seen by others.[63] In this fashion, communication not related to the focus of anger or fear may be influenced in such a way that others (and you) are confused.[64]

A second potentially damaging effect of hiding parts of yourself is that you cause apprehension in others. Suppose your employer tells you that you are failing to do your job adequately. You show no adverse reaction – you smile, remain calm, say nothing, and go on your way. Her interpretation is that you are a cool one, that you maintain your calmness through stiff self-disciplines, and do not easily get out of control. But she also wonders what you are not expressing; how many emotional stimuli do you take before you react; do you remain calm under stress until, at some point, you "break" and cannot be depended on at all? The point is this: you have given no way to assess your emotional behavior; people perceive only part of you and suspect there is more. People are confused and will be suspicious until they learn more about you, Interpersonal communication and personal relationships are distorted by attempts to hide parts of ourselves. Inauthentic behavior creates a façade of interpersonal communication while creating a disconnect more closely related to impersonal communication.

Often, people try to hide parts of their true selves by staying close to the "straight and narrow" ritualized patterns of interaction. They try to pursue only the "tried and true" forms of interpersonal behavior: "I can't receive negative feedback if I only do as everybody else does." The effect on the other person is one of appraising you as only a part-person – too cautious, too unnatural, and somewhat unreal. In some cases, the other person becomes apprehensive, wondering when your real self may show and what it will be like – and to what extent it may prove to be a threat.[65]

Dr. Jen's Rx

For...

Address..

R_x Date:.......................

The only way to attain one's ideal is to abandon one's illusions, but this is impossible unless you learn to separate the two.

Refills NA 1 2 3 4 5

Signature...

The second form of deceptive interaction is to pretend to be are something you are not. This approach includes attempts to communicate false messages about yourself – to wear masks or to erect facades.[66]

A number of points may be made about pretending to be what you are not. Firstly, pretending takes much energy and concentration; while focusing on your performance, you may miss clues as to the way people are actually perceiving you. Goffman makes the point that most people eventually discover that nobody is watching these performances and, in reality, those around you could not care less. Secondly, such playacting must be believable. Many television comedies have had a character pretending to be something he is not, with the the humor being that all others see through the façade. You may laugh at a comic character in a play, but you hardly want people laughing at your silly performance in real life.

Most people are incapable of carrying off deceptions on the nonverbal level. They signal their real feelings and attitudes through their muscular tension, changes of posture, facial expressions, jerky gestures, tone of voice, or other behaviors usually beyond their control.[67] Few people are adept at maintaining "poker faces" in their interactions. People may tolerate the pretense, but they usually recognize it for what it is.

Even when your pretenses win approval, the costs are great. Inside, you know you are a fraud; such self-knowledge is damaging to your self-esteem and eventually to your self-concept. Even if you use deception successfully in your interpersonal communication, you have only misused such interaction to defeat yourself. The person who won approval was a façade, and your real self goes unrecognized.

In the worst case, habitual pretending becomes a way of life. The more people pretend, the better they become at playing a part. And the better actor they become, the more they try to solve problems by pretense rather than by honestly facing issues and working out solutions based on reality. One phony bit of behavior thus produces another and, even if you convince others, you will be faced with the problem of trying to find your real self. "Who are you?" is the basic question asked of persons thought to be mentally disturbed. An unlimited pursuit of pretense in life has long been thought to produce the seeds of mental illness.[68] Authentic people hold realistic awareness of self and others and, possibly most difficult of all, are aware of the way others perceive them.

Authenticity and Conscience

Conscience is said to be the act of judging your behaviors by comparing them to the standards of your "idealized self," a moral judgment of your own conduct based upon the laws and customs of the society in which you have been reared.[69] It is a person's imaginative view of how he/she would like and ought to be.

In positive ways, consciences provide roadmaps for establishing socially conscious norms for behavior, and can be reinforced by threats of imprisonment, public disapproval, or terminated relationships. Unfortunately, strict conformity to some moral standards can sometimes force people to live in ways that endanger their mental and physical health.

If people have consciences based on a cruel and punitive morality, they may have exaggerated senses of duty that make them deny themselves legitimate pleasures. Thus, parents may deny themselves fun in life, insisting on a spartan existence in order to provide for their children. The necessity to repress anger, resentment, and temptation to pleasure may impose excessive stress on people and diminish their resistance to infectious diseases. The pressure caused by an overbearing morality is often found in persons with various forms of stress-related diseases, such as high blood pressure, heart diseases and possibly cancer.[70]

People's consciences may be viewed as unhealthy when:

1. They are excessively strict. Such people expect more of themselves, have a sterner morality and higher achievement goals, and feel much more guilt than their peers.

2. They have an authoritarian conscience. To disobey or question authority is wrong and synonymous with sin. This person becomes overwhelmed with guilt even at the thought of challenging vested authority.

3. Their consciences are repressed or projected. To repress is a refusal to think about something by resisting any mental processing. Such a person may have learned to refrain from making value judgments about his/her own behavior to avoid the painful experience of guilt. Projection occurs when a person transfers his or her own faults to another individual. These individuals perceive or "project" their own insecurities, ill will, or critical mindset. For example, cheating spouses are more likely to suspect their own spouses of cheating, whether there is reason to believe it or not. Overly critical individuals are more likely to believe that others are being critical of them. People with poor self-image, are more critical of others than people with higher self-esteem[71]

4. Their conscience is conflicted. In this case, one's ideals, values and taboos contradict one another. Conformity, when one value violates another value, results in guilt. For example, parents may have different standards for judging the behavior of their children. The mother may value obedience, submissiveness and gentleness; the father affirms assertive action, strength and aggressiveness. To please one parent is to displease the other. Some people attempt to resolve the conflicts by compartmentalizing their lives, as mentioned earlier. They may have one set of values at work, another at home, and another with peers, etc. Anxiety and added stress are consequences.

5. They harshly judge themselves and others by setting a ridiculously high standard that no one can achieve. When unrealistic perfectionist attitudes exist, individuals will always be deemed failures. Disappointments in self, others, and relationships will be common.

The joys of the present will never be fully realized as one is continually judging people and relationships to be inadequate compared to an ideal that exists only in fantasy.

A healthy conscience, conversely, will serve as a motivating factor toward personal growth, and makes decision-making simpler and consistent, since the person is being truthful to themselves. Being real and authentic in all eneavors leads to a healthy conscience. Such authenticity has the following salient attributes:

1. **Personal accessibility to consciousness**: A healthy conscience can be reflected upon. A person can formulate values, ideals, ethical precepts and taboos into words. This accessibility to consciences is important in the resolution of moral conflicts. If you are faced with a decision you can make your decision along moral lines much more readily when your ideals can be clearly stated. This doesn't mean you will always be thinking about your moral standards. You will respond to your conscience automatically; if you feel guilt, you recognize what aspects of your conscience have been violated and consider how to resolve this conflict. You have a moral compass.

2. **Self-affirmation**: A self-affirmed conscience is one in which you conform because you want to, not because you are afraid of disobeying. You have personally determined the rules by which you wish to live. The set of values, ideals and taboos that you have examined and affirmed become a part of your authentic self.

3. **Receptivity to questioning and change**: The healthy conscience is based upon general values and ideals that remain relatively fixed throughout life, but the behaviors these values call for may not be rigidly defined. As life circumstances change, some values may no longer be relevant. For example, a college student may feel certain luxuries are a waste of money and unnecessary, while the working professional may consider them reasonable acquisitions.

4. **Congruence with the social value system**: The person with a healthy conscience is living among other people, so will be obliged to share at least some of his/her ideals and taboos. This is not to say that his/her conscience will be absolutely congruent with social mores. They may find that their values are *more ethical* than the prevailing mores, so people will follow their conscience rather than the moral expectations of peers. People choose to leave homes and change churches and groups of friends rather than conforming to authoritarian demands.

Dealing with Conflict: Bridging the Great Divide

Since the founding of the USA, American citizens have not only tolerated but welcomed disagreements. Our democratic system of government was designed and built on values that encourage open exchange of ideas, willingness to formulate compromise, and willingness to put arguments to rest once a decision has been democratically reached. We as a country were unable to formulate any workable plan involving slavery, a practice that directly violated our stated belief that "All men are created equal." A civil war was the result.

Once more, our country is being tested as to our core values and our preference for a democratic society over an autocracy. We are again experiencing a "great divide." Close friends and families are being fractured by different realities. In addition to disagreeing over issues, Americans are disagreeing over facts.

As we seek to communicate with another (especially another with whom we disagree on some issue), we must establish a foundation on which we do agree – usually such agreement begins with facts, reality or shared perspective. For 350 years, educated, reasonable people have developed and utilized science and verified perceptions to create an objective truth, or "shared reality." "Scientific method" involves collecting data, reaching and testing conclusions and replicating studies to confirm the validity of conclusions reached. Scientific truth is a work in progress, with knowledge compounded, updated and corrected. Improved technology such as microscopes, x-rays, radar, photon generators, and computers greatly aid the process. Fortunately, dedicated scientists such as Galileo, Copernicus, Darwin, Curie, Freud, Einstein, and Hawking provided insights and data that changed the world's perception of reality. Scientific advances continue to change the world and our perception of it.

Science has been able to provide information and advance warnings of threats to our everchanging environment. We are able to witness the evidence of the world climate changes that are resulting in growing heat, an increase in the numbers and damage caused by natural disasters, and vanishing species of both animal and vegetation. The diversity of life enriches the quality of our lives in ways that are difficult to quantify; for example, the decline in honeybee populations is causing a loss of pollination for fruit crops and flowers.

Americans divide on numerous issues such as those in the following table. Consider the foundational truths that must be established for the two sides to enter into meaningful discussions:

48

Table 4.1 – Dividing Attitudes and Beliefs in U.S.

COLUMN A	COLUMN B
COVID-19 and Delta are health threats and we should respond accordingly.	COVID-19 and Delta aren't health threats. No need for masks/distancing.
Mandates are necessary to contain COVID-19 and Delta variant.	American personal freedoms are more important than passing requirements to wear masks or restricting free assembly.
Getting a COVID vaccine is essential. The cost of human lives it too much without vaccines.	Vaccines aren't necessary. Herd immunity will develop at some point.
Protest against police violence toward Black people is needed for change.	Civil protest breaks law and order.
America should seek cooperative relations with other nations.	America should come first at all times.
In the 2020 presidential election, Biden won.	In the 2020 presidential election, Trump won.
Voting rights should be provided and protected for all Americans.	The U.S. should legalize restrictions and barriers for minority voters.
U.S. should treat aliens humanely	Aliens should be banned.
Global warming is a fact with human action a major part of the cause.	If there is global warming, people are not responsible because the weather is always changing.
Abortions should be available to women who request them.	Abortions should be illegal.
Politicians' terms should be limited.	Politicians should be able to serve as many times as they are re-elected.
The American system is flawed but on the whole it incorporates checks and balances that allow it to work.	The system has been so badly corrupted by dirty politicians and bureaucrats that government cannot be trusted.

You can most likely add attitudes and actions to this list of dividing attitudes in the country. Many of these issues can be associated with one political party or the other.

On Wednesday, January 6, 2021, the United States Capitol was stormed during a violent riot and attack against the U.S. Congress, who were meeting to approve the results of the 2020 presidential election. Vice President Mike Pence was presiding over the Electoral College vote count as prescribed by the U.S. Constitution. In tweets, President Donald Trump had encouraged his supporters to come to Washington D.C. to his aid, to disrupt the joint session of Congress assembled to formalize Joe Biden's election. Among the tragic results were five deaths, at least 138 police officers injured, and an unknown number of rioters were hurt. Offices were vandalized, the building ransacked, property stolen and over $30 million was needed to repair the damage. Labeled an act of "domestic terrorism" by the FBI, opinion polls showed that a majority of Americans disapproved of the assault and Trump's involvement, but a sizable number of Republicans supported the attack, or at least did not blame Trump for it. [72]

Partisan tribalism seems to be the primary cause of vaccine reluctance and also disbelief in science is a tribal resistance, a marker of independence and strength. It demonstrates that "they" cannot tell "us" what to do. Many of these issues can be associated with one political party or the other. A democracy cannot long endure if a majority of citizens support their allegiance to a political party over the welfare of the nation.

In order to better understand the great divide of United States citizenry, Oprah Winfrey called together a politically diverse group of individuals from the Grand Rapids area to discuss their views on politics in August, 2017 and the lively discussion aired on a segment on 60 Minutes entitled, "Division (September, 2017)." The discussion was so interesting, that another meeting of the same participants convened the following February. The meeting consisted of animated discussions with voices frequently overlapping. At one point, several participants admitted that they feared a civil war was imminent. Despite the amount of disagreement, the group stayed in touch, became friends, organized outings and connected frequently as a private Facebook chat group they called "America's Hope".[73] They even attended a town hall meeting together. The pollster stated that conversations such as the one she moderated "stopped happening in this country more than a year ago." As he continued: "When it became dangerous to tell people in the so-called fly-over-states that you supported Hillary Clinton; when it became dangerous to tell people in New York or L.A. that you supported Donald Trump, they were afraid for their friendships; they were afraid at work and so we just stopped talking politics." [74]

While the members did not sway others to their side on issues, something important occurred according to the moderator, "…they came to respect each other, appreciate each other, and live each other's lives to some degree so that they could empathize." During the conversations group members agreed that the politicians in Washington needed to talk with each other as this group had. One participant said, "I really, really like these people." And another asserted "…what changed for me, the hope (of common ground) became a reality." And a third panelist commented, "That's America – you have the liberty to agree to disagree. You shouldn't take that away." [75] The simple act of discussion allowed these people to drop stereotypes, and avoid tribalistic tendencies, and though they didn't always reach agreement, they were not afraid to voice their opinions and they listened to one another respectfully. One participant summarized the divide outside the panel this way "…we're not actually listening and understanding each other, and that's causing the divide." [76]

A key problem is the absence of a societal agreement on the existence of truth and reality. By "truth" we mean the kind of conclusion a trial jury or committee of inquiry is designed to handle. Reality exists whether people are there to witness it or not. Actions and events actually occur, such as the events on January 6. Scientific truth is based on common sense, logic and critical reasoning. Scientists do make mistakes and print erroneous conclusions, but science welcomes replication and corrects the errors as the search for truth continues. People's ability to perceive has been greatly enhanced by technology, medicine, mathematical sophistication, and logic. Conversely, just because a lot of people believe it, doesn't make it true.

The Threat of Conspiracy Theories

Conspiracy theories have circulated for years. Every time a U.S. President dies in office, causation is linked to conspiracy, particularly in the case of John F. Kennedy. The moon landing, the 9/11 attack, the existence of "the deep state," or government cover-ups of findings of UFO's have prompted conspiracy theories. Harm occurs when conspiracy-theory-believers become disconnected from shared reality. If people believe COVID-19 is a hoax, they are not likely to engage in best practices such as social distancing, mask wearing, vaccinations, or hand-washing, resulting in risk of spreading the virus. As more conspiracy theories are accepted, believers start to distrust institutions, scientists, people in roles of authority or power. They find more conspiracy theories to believe, and detach themselves even more from shared reality.[77]

Another factor that drives conspiracy beliefs is group attachment. Political parties provide a "tribe that has our back" and influences our beliefs. When trusted leaders promote conspiracy theories, those theories undergo less scrutiny than if they are presented from unknown sources.

A phenomenon that demonstrates the willingness of many Americans to believe and promote conspiracy theories is the COVID-19 crisis. Political scientist Joseph Uscinski at the University of Miami has defined a conspiracy theory as: "An accusatory perception in which a small group of powerful people is acting in secret for their own benefit against the common good – and in a way that undermines our bedrock ground rules against the wide-spread use of force and fraud. In addition, this theory hasn't been found to be true by the appropriate experts, using data and evidence that is available for anyone to refute."[78]

Among the numerous conspiracy theories about COVID-19 is that when vaccine is injected into a person, a microchip is implanted that permits the government to track the recipient. As Professor Uscinski mentions: "Some think that Big Pharma is behind the COVID-19 'scam,' and they're going to make money by selling us a phony vaccine for a phony disease." [79]

Some of the theories suggest that Bill Gates, the Koch brothers, George Soros, or 5G technology are responsible for spreading the virus. A poll in 2020 found 29 percent of Americans believe that the disease was exaggerated for political gain to hurt Donald Trump in the election of 2020. A similar number thought it was some sort of bioweapon that spread the disease on purpose.

A group calling themselves Q-Anon spread misinformation about COVID-19 and conspiracy theories, based upon a set of bizarre and extreme beliefs. Followers believed that Donald Trump was fighting the "deep state," which they said is composed of satanic pedophiles and human traffickers. Q-Anon believed that some celebrities and politicians enjoyed feasting on babies, and drinking their blood. Fortunately, the number of people continuing to support Q-Anon is said to be diminishing. [80]

Q-Anon was still able to attract several hundred followers to Dealey Plaza, the site of John F. Kennedy's assassination in Dallas, Texas on November 2. 2021, the Anniversary of the event. The group had promised that "John F. Kennedy, Jr. (who died in a plane crash in 1999 at the age of 38) would come back to life and appear to begin the reinstatement of Donald Trump as president."[81] Disappointingly for the crowd, he did not make an appearance.

Our freedoms in the U.S., such as speech and religion, must be protected. Like the people of Grand Rapids, we must continue to discuss, debate, listen, and analyze issues. Listening before arguing indicates respect and a willingness to overcome impersonal discourse. As we listen, respect and react to individuals in a personal fashion, differences become less important and people become more important. As we train ourselves to face our fears, give up our stereotypes, reflect on our automatic responses, and choose healthy responses we strengthen ourselves, our relationships and our society.

Personal Reflection

Evaluate your own conscience. Where do you place yourself on a line from unhealthy to healthy on the attributes cited in this chapter? Who or what has had the greatest influence on your values and ideals?

Chapter 5 - Reciprocal Self-Disclosure in a Healthy Relationship

Next to the death penalty, the most severe punishment that can be inflicted upon a person is solitary confinement. This deprives the incarcerated of human company, companionship and communication so that they have no one to talk to or to share life with. They are dehumanized because people need one another to be human. Enforced solitude may, in extreme cases, lead to mental illness, extreme stress and loss of motivation to live. Unfortunately, there are many kinds of self-inflicted solitude that create a similar kind of distress.

In some American families, the members function primarily in roles that create distance between one another. Sometimes families divide themselves whether traditionally or untraditionally into roles such as "the provider," "the peace maker," "the go-between," "the black sheep." Their interactions become locked in impersonal interactions as if they are strangers to one another. Regrettably, they do not discuss personal and private matters with each other.

Similarly, relationships with close friends can reach a standstill if true feelings are withheld. It is in the intimacy of our personal communication and the sharing of core emotions and ideas that we can develop growing relationships with others, including family members. This openness provides the basis for healthy communication – the capacity to be authentic in relationships.

In this chapter, a set of criteria will be provided by which you can evaluate relationships with family members and close friends to discern if they diminish or promote one's personal health.

Basic Interpersonal Needs

The old adage that "people need people" has long been accepted. A logical follow-up question is "In what ways do people need people?" Just as nonfulfillment of a biological need leads to physical illness and sometimes death, so too does denial of an interpersonal need. Unsatisfactory personal relationships lead directly to difficulties associated with emotional illness and general loss of motivation. William C. Schutz in the 1960's identified the three basic needs that provide a conceptual system for the analysis, prediction and explanation for human behavior.[82]

1. **Inclusion.** This need requires satisfactory interactions regarding feelings of mutual interest. This social need is to feel that people include me, are interested in me, and feel that I am interested in them. The healthy outcome of inclusion is feeling that I am significant and accepted. Demanding too much inclusion can lead to feeling suffocated. On the other hand, results of exclusion can lead to feeling insignificant and unrecognized. The extreme absence of inclusive fulfillment leads to severe mood disorders.

2. **Control**. Everyone needs to feel that their behaviors can result in predictable and meaningful outcomes. The interpersonal need for control is defined behaviorally as the need to establish and maintain a satisfying relationship with respect to power. Healthy outcomes are balanced, reciprocal and democratic, giving and receiving respect. Unhealthy outcomes based on an absence of trust and respect, force individuals into roles of opposition such as autocrat/rebel, or dictator/ submissive. Without control people can feel incompetent, powerless, stupid, and irresponsible. Unhealthy pursuits of control can lead to impersonal responses, bullying, game playing, and passive aggression. Extreme cases result in psychopathic, obsessive-compulsive reactions. Personal control will be discussed later as it relates to empowerment

3. **Affection**. Everyone needs to establish and maintain a feeling of mutual affection with others. We need to feel that we are lovable and able to love others to a mutually satisfying degree. People must truly "see" us for who we are, be friendly, and demonstrate that they like us. Unhealthy over- or under-personal actions reflect dislike, and we tend to feel no good and unlovable. In extreme cases individuals become neurotic. Unhealthy responses to these three basic needs are anxiety, hostility and ambivalence.

Think back over your interactions with others during the last day or two. What impresses you most about the way you and other people seemed to get along, relate to each other, or feel about one another? The presence of the 2020 pandemic threat introduced, for most, a new significant variable to our social interaction. Nonverbal actions were affected by prohibitions on touch, facial coverings like masks and bandanas, and distance requirements. "Social distancing "immediately eliminated the support we feel from the touch of a friend.

You may recall that someone was angry with you or appeared to be. You may also recall someone showed you kindness, tenderness, affection – especially if you felt yourself responding in a similar way. It could be that someone tried to dominate you, tried to "push you around," or "put you down." Maybe someone responded readily to your suggestions, seemed to want your advice, or tried to do things the way you like to see them done. You may have difficulty recalling someone who seemed to be avoiding you or wanted to be left alone – they may have been so successful that you did not notice their avoidance behavior. On the other hand, you likely recall with ease someone who seemed especially interested in talking with you, a person with whom you interact frequently or for extended periods.

The degree of involvement in a human relationship refers not only to the amount of interaction between the participants, but also to the importance each attaches to the interaction. If two people seldom see or talk to each other, and when they do, they simply exchange impersonal greetings, the degree of their mutual involvement with each other is small. For example, you may have a co-worker who ordinarily sits on the opposite side of the room. Did he attend work yesterday? If you can't remember, your degree of *involvement* in this relationship is low, even if you tend to see and talk to him two or three times a week. Conversely, you and your father may live in different cities, see each other twice a year, and communicate only four or five times a year, but still have a high degree of *involvement* in your relationship. If each idea he presents and each sentence he speaks or writes, is given careful thought and attention, then your degree of *involvement* is high.

The degree of *involvement* is closely related to the amount of personal information exchanged. If your *involvement* with another person is to be high, you and that person will need to reveal significant parts of yourselves to each other. Research data show that when self-disclosure is high, interpersonal *involvement* is increased.

Suppose, for example, that you meet someone on the tennis courts. You like his looks. This initiates a degree of *involvement* on your part. You chat a while and you like the sense of personal values implied by the conversation: he expresses loyalty to school, regard for friends, and appreciation of personal skill and achievement. You play tennis for an hour and receive impressions of honesty in keeping score, determination to do one's best, and fairness in judging out-of-bounds serves. At lunch, you are impressed by his courtesy and consideration for others, cleanliness in eating habits, and friendliness in meeting your needs or wishes. During the next half-hour, you hear of his hopes for graduation, ambition to be a pediatrician, frustration over required courses, and sadness over the recent loss of a grandfather. If over the ensuing days such self-disclosure continues, and you continue to be interested in such personal information, *involvement* in the relationship will increase. In addition, disclosure of the way he *feels* about *you* can lead to greater involvement. If he shows you the way he feels regarding your hopes, ambitions, values and frustrations, your degree of *involvement* will be heightened, and the relationship will be of greater importance, both to you and to the other person.

As people interact and disclose personal information to each other, they tend to reach little agreements on what is important and what is not. Out of this sharing comes a working consensus of mutual empathy and consideration. There is also a tendency to close the gaps between their individual differences of opinion. In essence, *involvement* in a relationship means that participants interact in ways that are important to each other. As *involvement* is increased, the other two dimensions of a relationship become important: *control* and *affection*. In an established relationship, the degree of involvement is usually quite stable. The amount of interaction may vary from day to day, but such variations are expected and routine. In such a relationship, control and affection are then of greatest concern.

Let's suppose that you are a young woman and you meet a man you do not know. As you are introduced and start to get acquainted, you find him attractive. He shows warmth and friendliness – even potential affection. In addition, he tends to dominate your conversation and insists that he take you to lunch. You are resistant to being led or pushed, particularly with a new acquaintance. On the other hand, your resistance has somewhat cooled your relationships with other men previously, and now you appreciate signs of male friendliness and affection.

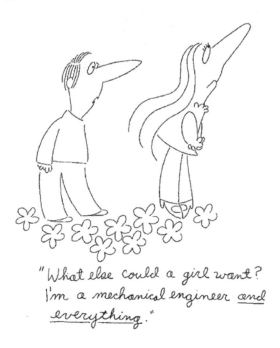

"What else could a girl want? I'm a mechanical engineer and everything."

We can tentatively predict that you and your new acquaintance will engage in a friendly power struggle. In addition, you will be somewhat torn between wanting to accept his friendly attention and resisting his domination. You may insist on paying for your own lunch, but hope he will ask you to dinner. Your power struggle may terminate the relationship, if either of you tire of the required effort. Alternatively, the friendly warmth and affection may keep the relationship going; and the two of you may find ways of sharing power or influence over each other. Perhaps you may allow yourself to be dominated only in ways that don't threaten your personhood or self-esteem.

Note that we have said little about where you go together or what you do. What matters most in a relationship is the degrees of domination of one over the other and the emotional tone of your feelings – the degrees of dominance/submission and affection/hostility.

In a relationship, affectionate behavior on the part of one person tends to produce affectionate responses on the part of the other; likewise, hostile behavior tends to produce hostility. We may thus conclude that *interpersonal behavior characterized along the bipolar dimension of affection/hostility ordinarily elicits similar responses.* Unlike affection/ hostility, dominant behavior in a relationship tends to produce submissive responses. This, of course, is true only if interaction continues. If dominant behavior by one person is continued and resistance is shown by the other person, the relationship may be terminated. If a relationship is continued in which a power struggle occurs, this struggle may last for days, months, or even years. In some families, it may never be resolved; it may lead to use of manipulative games or strategies that continue endlessly. Concerning power, it is interesting to note that while the appetite for sex or comfort is limited, the appetite for power can be limitless.

Submissive behavior in a relationship tends to elicit domination by the other person. If you are dominated, it is not entirely the other person's fault. Submission reinforces dominating behavior, and vice versa. We may thus state a second principle of interpersonal behavior in action: *behavior that may be characterized along the bipolar dimension of dominance/submission tends to elicit reciprocal behavior; dominance reinforces submission; submission reinforces dominance.*

Let's turn our attention once again to the imaginary relationship previously discussed; you, a young woman, warmly interacting with a young man who attempts to dominate you in a friendly way. Let us suppose that the interpersonal warmth continues and the attempts to dominate largely subside. As you and he interact, your interpersonal behavior, as well as his, can largely be explained and predicted in terms of the two principles cited above: affection or hostility tend to elicit *similar* responses, and dominance or submissiveness tend to elicit *reciprocal* responses. As you and he continue to interact, your behavior produces responses by him; these responses, in turn, produce responses by you.

 Reflect on several of your relationships: parent-child, boss-employee, close friend. How healthy are they? What role does power play?

Unhealthy Relationship 'Games'

In his popular 1960's book *Games People Play,* the late Eric Berne analyzed relationship patterns in terms of "games".[83] The term *game,* however, is somewhat misleading. Typically, a game implies two sides who follow mutually agreeable and coordinated sets of rules. Berne's games tend to operate as the victimization of one party by the other party through fraudulent, manipulative means.

A typical game as analyzed by Berne was one he called *Corner.* According to Berne *cornering* consists of a delayed refusal to follow another's ploy to produce a show of affection. In this game, a wife suggests to her spouse that they go to a movie; the spouse agrees. The wife makes a comment that maybe they shouldn't because the house needs painting. They have previously agreed that they don't have the money to paint the house right now; therefore, this is not a "reasonable" time to relate such an expensive consideration to the price of a movie. The spouse responds rudely to the house-painting remark. The wife suggests that her spouse should go alone. This is the critical artificial ploy of the game. The spouse knows very well from past experiences this suggestion is not to be taken seriously. What the wife really wants is to be "honeyed up" and told everything will be all right. But the spouse refuses to show her this affectionate attention. The spouse leaves, feeling relieved but abused; the wife is left feeling resentful. In this instance, the spouse won this game because all he did was to do as she suggested – literally. Berne's conclusion is: "They both know this is cheating but, since she said it, she is cornered." This is a cruel game played to achieve a *show* of affection; its target is manipulation or control of another person, and its interpersonal attitude beneath the surface – no matter who wins – is not affection but hostility. There are many games that can be played in relationships. When the purpose is to manipulate others, the result is unhealthy. Rather than garnering love affection, admiration, and respect, games tend to generate hostility, resentment, separation, and loathing.

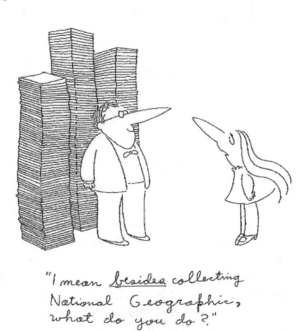

"I mean *besides* collecting National Geographics, what do you do?"

Characteristics of Relationships That Promote Good Health

The following three characteristics describe relationships between two people that engender health, growth, and well-being in both parties:

1. **Authenticity**: The two people communicate authentically with one another and are able to share each other's perspective. The only way for people to truly know one another is through mutual self-disclosure. The two people make their subjective worlds known to each other in a back and forth, continuing dialogue. Mutual trust is established.

2. **Reasonable demands upon one another**: Their demands and claims upon one another are reasonable. The demands that each partner imposes on the other as conditions for the continuation of the relationship are realistic, mutually agreed upon, and consistent with the values of the other. They are actively concerned with one another's growth and happiness, value the autonomy of the other and, further, wants the partner to do what he/she wants to do.

Dr. Jen's Rx

For.........

Address.........

R_X Date:.........

Openness is greatest in childhood, when we are being defined and validated.

Refills NA 1 2 3 4 5

Signature.........

3. **Freedom from control**: Each person treasures the freedom of the other to be himself/herself and does not try to control the other. They do not try to change one another through manipulation, yet can openly express any wishes for changes in the other. There is no question that we can change another person by manipulation, coercion, force, threats and "brainwashing." While such tactics will be effective in the short run, they will usually be achieved at the cost of resentment and hostility toward the person dictating the terms. The overbearing parent or teacher rarely considers the other person's needs and values.

The "victim" will rebel and terminate the relationship when possible. When manipulation becomes a pattern of interacting with others, it is a sign of impaired relational health, based upon distrust, a repression of spontaneous feelings and overt deception.[84]

Dr. Jen's Rx

For...

Address...

R_X Date:.......................

The most fatiguing activity in the world is the drive to seem other than you are; it is far less exhausting to become what you want to be than to maintain this pretense.

Refills NA 1 2 3 4 5

Signature...

Developing Self-Disclosure Skills

Self-disclosure is difficult for many people. If a family doesn't talk about personal feelings, such communication is new and threatening. Understanding the importance of talking honestly with significant others is crucial to developing depth, trust and self-acceptance.

Self-disclosers are more self-content, more competent and adaptive, more perceptive, more extroverted, and more trusting and positive toward others than non-disclosing persons. A positive cycle develops as disclosure promotes positive regard, and such regard leads to deeper disclosures when reciprocated. Data from therapy, self-help groups, and clinical research suggest that sharing your emotions helps prevent disease, improves your general health, and lessens psychological problems.[85]

What are the topics you're willing to discuss with someone you like and trust? What are the personal feelings and topics that you keep hidden? All of us have secrets, but we tend to conceal so much that is unnecessary. How comfortable are you with self-disclosure? On what topics do you feel transparent with trusted others and what topics make you feel guarded? Consider such topics as:

- **Attitudes and personal opinions** – The kind of people I like and dislike, political opinions, sexual feelings, my values, and religious feelings.

- **Relationships** – How I'm getting along with my spouse, children, and people I care about . . . people with whom I enjoy socializing and being together; the enjoyment of my friends and people upon whom I rely.
- **Personal interest**. What social activities do I truly enjoy; what do I do for fun; my favorite food, music, TV shows and movies?
- **Economics and well-being**. What are my career ambitions, my successes and failures, my economic needs and comfort level? How do I feel about my salary and working position?
- **Personality**. What do I affirm about myself, my strengths and my weaknesses? Do I have personal problems such as uncontrolled emotions or moodiness?
- **Physical issues**. Am I concerned about my health? Am I satisfied with my appearance, my body parts, my fitness?

In early stages of a relationship people characteristically engage in "small talk" as they become acquainted with one another. As their comfort level and mutual trust grow, they begin to talk about more serious ideas. When people find that they feel satisfaction from sharing ideas, opinions and feelings, the relationship deepens and friendship develops.

Scholars have presented four guidelines for self-disclosure that can build and sustain healthy relationships.[86] Self-disclose the kind of information you want others to disclose to you. Reciprocity is important.

1. Self-disclose more intimate information only when the disclosure represents an acceptable risk.
2. Continue intimate self-disclosure only if it is reciprocated.
3. Move self-disclosure to deeper levels gradually.
4. Reserve personal sensitive self-disclosures for ongoing intimate relationships.

Dr. Jen's Rx

For...

Address...

Rx

Date:.......................

*The more a person is open and
transparent, the greater the possibility to
learn new self-definitions and improve
self-concept, possibly the single most
important factor affecting human
behavior.*

Refills NA 1 2 3 4 5

Signature..

The Importance of Reciprocity and Feedback

When you are engaged in a session of self-disclosure, you must be authentically as interested in the other person's feelings, problems and opinions as you are in expressing yours. By the mutual interaction, each party learns what appropriate disclosure is. The danger of unbalanced reciprocity is that we may under-disclose or over-disclose.

Considerable research has shown that women disclose more to strangers and new acquaintances than men. Men are comfortable talking about external topics such as the weather, team sports scores, or politics while women are more likely to discuss feelings and personal topics. Women tend to disclose material that is personal, feeling-oriented, and may involve negative emotions. Men, on the other hand, more readily disclose information that is factual and relatively neutral or positive in emotional tone.[87]

It should not be assumed that the sheer amount of self-disclosure between the parties in a relationship is an index to the health of the relationship or of the persons. Factors such as timing, interest level of the other person, feedback indicating appropriateness, and the effects of the disclosures upon the parties involved must be considered. Sidney Jourard suggested that too much disclosure as well as too little disclosure is associated with unhealthy communication, whereas a healthy middle ground met under appropriate conditions and settings is desirable. As a general principle, he suggested that people who feel obliged to lie to others about their inner being are making themselves sick, asserting "We may find that those who become sick most frequently, physically and mentally, have long been downright liars to others and to themselves."[88]

As you might expect, the use of and levels of self-disclosure differ from culture to culture. Americans tend to disclose more about themselves than people from most other cultures. In the beginning stages of a cross-cultural friendship the cultural differences can lead to misunderstandings and discomfort. For example, a person from the U.S. might think that a new acquaintance from an Eastern culture is "stand offish" when they seem reluctant to discuss personal feelings, or seeking more personal space. Regardless of these cultural differences, researchers discovered that, across culture, when relationships become more intimate, self-disclosure increases.[89] In addition, the researchers found that the more partners disclosed to each other, the more they were attracted to one another.

How do we know what is appropriate disclosure? The key is both verbal and nonverbal response to our disclosures. Does your partner show genuine interest, caring and self-disclosure in return? It takes emotional intelligence to know what an acceptable moderation of disclosures is and when a friend is ready for deeper interactions.

There are, of course, dangers in self-disclosure. You may upset the other person, or lose their friendship, and there is the risk that your disclosure may be revealed or used against you. That is why disclosing to a trusted individual, noting feedback and receiving reciprocity are crucial to healthy communication.

Isolation and Abusive Relationships

As the world's families were forced to isolate themselves for much of 2020 due to the COVID-19 crisis, the slogan "Safe at Home" was not true for everyone. The "stay at home" orders gravely impacted intimate partner violence and child abuse. Before this pandemic, a victim could flee a violent situation by going to another family member, a friend, a shelter, or other sites that offered protection. With everyone at home, victims of abuse had no place to escape.[90]

The director of the organization, The Network: Advocating Against Domestic Violence based in Chicago stated that "Victims and the abusers have to stay at the scene of the crime." The Network runs a 24-hour hotline, statewide that saw a thirty percent increase in the number of calls when the initial confinement order went into effect. The coronavirus was cited as a cause of the abuse. Abusers were preventing their partners from going to their jobs, blocking them from needed healthcare service, and keeping them from accessing safety tools like gloves, masks, or sanitizers. [91]

In addition to intimate partner violence, concerns were also raised about child abuse. The pandemic increased stress levels of parents in a multitude of ways. Financial strains were increased as the economy waned. Families were cooped up in their homes. Everyone was separated from friends and support systems.

Children had fewer outlets for expending energy. Tempers flared. Parents found it more difficult to deal with children's aggression and misbehavior. Behavioral disorders became even more difficult to tolerate. Opportunities to remove oneself from volatile situations were decreased. Abused children were in even greater peril than prior to the pandemic as they experienced limited contact with teachers and school counselors who could identify signs of abuse and report to proper authorities.

Regardless of age, self-disclosure with a trusted person is crucial to one's mental and physical well-being. Healthy relationships take time and energy, both of which are in limited supply, so you must be selective when determining which relationships deserve your priority. Initiating a communicative style based on openness, acceptance, and honesty will promote a climate of trust and reciprocity.

Personal Reflections

1. Look over the list of topics suggested in this chapter. Evaluate your level of disclosure with a significant other. Analyze one another's level of sharing. Are you mutually comfortable with the depth and reciprocity of disclosures?

2. Analyze an on-going significant relationship. How are issues of decision-making handled? Do you sense any manipulation generated from either party?

Chapter 6 - Trust, Confidence and Societal Health

Authentic communication is crucial to the health of society and all communicators. If you cannot accurately discern the truth, it is easy to be victimized. By hiding your real self behind a constructed facade, your feelings of inadequacy, fear of rejection, and lack of self-awareness can interfere with your healthy behavior within society. Healthy communicators experience the freedom of open self-expression, and those who find themselves in their presence benefit from it.

Without trust, all human interactions would be suspect. All social engagements, including marriage, are dependent on confidence in future behaviors based on past trustworthy behaviors. Lives and livelihoods are at risk if trust is misplaced.

The Problems Caused by Scams and Untruths

All lives have been negatively affected by deception, scams and untruths. Consider the true story of Patricia C., who spent nearly $200,000 for taxes and insurance to claim a sweepstakes prize she never received. The contest representative telephoned 83-year-old Patricia, sometimes treating her like a best friend, and other times threatening her. He even mailed her an invoice for $25,830 in past-due payments.

Patricia, who had no mental incapacities, saw contest reps as her *allies*, while regarding her relatives as those trying to *interfere* with her becoming rich. An expert associated with the AARP said, "For scam victims to admit they were wrong means they're stupid and unable to take care of themselves."[92] When protectors take over finances or lecture victims about their mistakes, it plays right into the scammers' hands by threatening the target's independence.

The Federal Trade Commission received more than 400,000 complaints about computer fraud in 2016, costing consumers a total of $744 million. Scams included requesting advance payments for credit service, foreign money offers, investment opportunities, mortgage foreclosure relief, "free prizes," and false tax billings among countless others. Frauds invade our lives through the internet, in person, and by phone. In 2016 some 77 percent of all scams were conducted by phone. Consumers fall prey to scams in which con-artists pretend to be someone trustworthy, such as a government official or a service technician, to fraudulently seek money. Older Americans are most vulnerable.[93] Our failure to be authentic with one another and our inability to detect deception have created an atmosphere of distrust. When our phones ring, what are the chances that it is a Robo-call, or a scam aimed at defrauding us of money?

Because of international events, many of us feel that we are living in particularly perilous times, times of increased distrust, lies and deception. The specter of nuclear war never fully disappeared. While most Americans believe that nuclear war is highly unlikely, a majority also believe that America should continue to build new and better nuclear weapons. Such contradictory attitudes and the resulting behaviors are unhealthy on many levels.

Various aspects of our society appear to be contributing to the problem. For many, our democratic values appear to be eroding and many people are suspect of government in general. Recent polls show that the majority of U.S. citizens do not trust elected officials. A cynical and suspicious attitude toward our government and its legislative members runs deeply throughout our citizenry, including suspicions about government collusion with Russia to undermine our elections and democracy This attitude is reciprocated by the government during the Trump presidency when it frequently voiced profound distrust of citizens and the press. Fears were rampant as the government threatened to deport immigrants and migrants, and suppress freedoms of minority communities such as Muslims, LGBTQs and black people.

Dr. Jen's Rx

For..

Address...

R_x Date:...........................

Negative experiences, as well as positive experiences, have a lasting impact.

Refills NA   1   2   3   4   5

Signature...

Lies, deceit, surveillance, and imprisonment of dissenters have all been tools to control the populace. An "us versus them" mentality has been cultivated, adding to the environment of distrust and fear. The cover of *TIME* magazine on April 3, 2017, even raised the question, "Is Truth Dead?" Being lied to or misled makes us vulnerable to bad decisions and relationships and, thus, subjects us to victimization.

Economically, our country's situation is puzzling. As the wealthiest nation in the world, we are unable to agree on how to provide for all our people. Recently, the effort and programs to reduce and manage poverty have been eliminated, while the top one percent of our populace receives more income than the bottom 50 percent, and the divide has continued to grow. As the gap between rich and poor in this country widens, also does the gap between rich countries and poor countries. This could be evidenced recently as wealthy countries developed and controlled how vaccines for COVID-19 were dispersed.

Large corporations and Wall Street have an inordinate influence on our government and on our lives. High office continues to go predominately to white men of wealth. For example, all but three of Donald Trump's cabinet were millionaires and, at the same time, over half of our 116th Congress (officials elected to represent all American citizens) were millionaires. *Forbes* magazine reports that Biden's 2021 15-member cabinet consists of thirteen millionaires or multi-millionaires with a net worth of around $118 million. Trump's cabinet was worth $6.2 billion and contained seventeen millionaires, two multimillionaires, and a billionaire. It is obvious that the wealthy elite continue to determine the destinies of middle and lower economic class individuals.[94]

White men are 30 percent of U.S. population but 62 percent of office holders. Women are 51 percent of the population but fill only 31 percent of political offices. Meanwhile, people of color make up 40 percent of the US population and only 13 percent of office holders.

Violence has been a constant in our society. The ready availability of guns makes daily killings in most cities a routine occurrence. In large cities, people double- and triple-lock their doors. Walking on streets at night has become a hazardous activity in many areas.

There are many theories regarding the causes of wide-spread violence. While the authors don't pretend to be experts in this field, we do offer two factors that are discussed in this book: first, random violence rarely occurs when each individual feels he/she is included in an ongoing, purposeful process. For humans, it is fundamental to be a part of a group or society. When members become alienated from the mainstream of society, the climate is set for impersonal or random violence to be rampant. The second point is that, for such violence to occur, the belief in the worth, dignity, or rights of the victims are disregarded. Hate for the "other" takes precedence over empathy or guilt. Consider these two factors and how they may have influenced police shootings, riots and terrorist attacks.

Not only is it important to be authentic, but it is important to encourage others to be their authentic selves and to accept those who are different from us. An American Psychological Association survey revealed that 24 percent of the general population polled by the APA reported that they experienced unfair treatment or discrimination on a day-to-day basis, and three in ten of those individuals said they changed their behavior or appearance to avoid harassment.

Some of the populations that experience increased stress levels include the following: lesbians, gays, bisexuals, transgenders and teenagers. The poll also indicated that the higher the stress levels, the poorer physical health reported by participants.[95] A survey of more than 7,000 transgender people conducted by the National Center for Transgender Equality and the National Gay and Lesbian Task Force released in 2010, found that 41 percent of transgender people in the U.S. attempted to commit suicide that year, 19 percent reported being refused medical care because of their gender-nonconforming status, and 2 percent were violently assaulted in a doctor's office.[96] In an article in the journal *Psychological Bulletin*, Ian Meyer of Columbia University identified "minority stress" as a factor in the higher prevalence of mental disorders in lesbian, gay and bisexual people; he goes on to explain that "stigma, prejudice and discrimination create a hostile and stressful social environment that causes mental health problems."[97] Hopefully with new laws, conditions are changing.

The recent violence and bullying in our culture makes it unsurprising that there has been a steady stream toward abandoning personal freedoms and permitting more authoritarian control. In subsequent chapters, we will suggest ways to empower ourselves and our leaders and restore faith in the democratic system without seeking authoritarian means.

Rise in Fraud and Scams During the 2020 Pandemic

The COVID-19 outbreak in 2020 created pain on a societal level. As CNN reported: "Russian state media and pro-Kremlin outlets are waging a disinformation campaign about the pandemic to sow 'panic and fear' in the west." The aim of the disinformation was to aggravate the public health crisis in western countries by undermining public trust in the national health care systems.[98] Misinformation and lies on social media have continued to slow our progress against the pandemic.

In the U.S., the Justice Department created a central fraud hotline (1-866-720-5721). *Time* reported that marketing schemers quickly began to offer "senior care packages" that included a hand sanitizer and even a purported vaccine that didn't exist.[99] Hate groups sent anti-Semitic messages that Jews were somehow responsible for the pandemic and some extreme hate groups suggested tainting doorknobs with the virus to cause FBI and police officers to contract the illness.

Hundreds of masks were stolen in Oregon amid the shortage for health care workers. A Missouri man was coughing in a store, and told the store clerks he had a high fever before threatening them with the disease. Similar incidents were reported in Illinois and Pennsylvania.[100]

New York officials ordered *The Jim Bakker Show* (known for his televangelist high jinks in the 1980's) to stop marketing "colloidal silver products" as a cure for the coronavirus. The World Health Organization had stated that no specific medicine has been yet discovered to prevent or treat the disease.[101]

Con artists peddled fake COVID-19 cures and financial scams around the world. In Uganda, parliament speaker Rebecca Kadaga endorsed a chemical that a businessman had discovered and wanted produced for the world market. The company that was preparing the product revealed that it was actually a disinfectant that is not to be ingested. Two weeks later, the president of the U.S. raised a similar suggestion before claiming a day later that it had been done in jest.

A Kenyan clinic sold false testing kits and other fraudsters offered contaminated banknotes at a large discount in South Africa. Fraudsters in the United Kingdom tried to scam people to buy medical supplies online, targeting people who were increasingly isolated at home and vulnerable.[102] We all need the ability to sort reality and truth from fiction and lies.

Problems Caused by Disinformation, Deceptions and Public Toleration of Untruths

Until the past decade, our country had no concept of the massively dangerous destructive powers of misinformation to our well-being. U.S. General Stanley McChrystal, the leader of all U.S. military operations in Afghanistan, retired when the U.S. withdrew. A TIME reporter, Belinda Luscombe, interviewed him and asked the general, what did he consider to be the biggest threat "America must face down." He responded, neither the Taliban nor a global pandemic. It's disinformation, or – as he calls it "…the ability to pollute our consciousness." The hidden threat of deception is not just that people will believe the wrong thing, but that they will start to think the wrong way. False information can be corrected, but "if you change the way I think, the logic process I go through, then you've changed a cultural part of society." Disinformation, he says, has "the potential and the power of weapons of mass destruction."[103]

Your Sense of Reality

Your chances of behaving in a healthy way are increased if you perceive the world accurately and form your beliefs from these accurate perceptions. But we know that unfulfilled needs and strong emotions can so influence experiences that facts become misinterpreted, flawed conclusions reached, and, truths overlooked. One political consultant reportedly said during the 2016 presidential campaign, "Why look for the truth when we can easily create it?" Such attitudes resulted in the introduction of the phrase, "alternative facts". The 2016 New Word of the Year, according to the Oxford Dictionary, was, "post-truth," which they define as "an adjective relating to circumstances in which objective facts are less influential in shaping public opinion than emotional appeal," These new terms reflected an ominous shift in Western politics. Truth was no longer based on verifiable evidence, but on whatever a strong leader said it was.

Let's consider a personal example of reality testing. One of our aging relatives sought help with a problem she was having. She believed her apartment-mate in the retirement home was stealing her money, jewelry, and even stationery. She noticed various items missing from her dresser from time to time, and she concluded her apartment-mate was guilty. However, she did not confront the woman with the allegations; instead, she felt distrust, resentment and discomfort as she struggled to keep these feelings to herself. Their relationship deteriorated into one of formality, silence, forced politeness and false expressions of friendship.

We asked why she didn't bring the issue up with her apartment-mate. She said that if she did so, her mate would hate her, and she couldn't stand that. When asked if there could be any other explanation for the loss, she couldn't think of any. We suggested that her mate may be bothered and saddened by the way their relationship had deteriorated and would welcome some frank talk to settle things. She reluctantly agreed to broach the subject.

When we saw her next, she was happy to report that the two had discussed the whole incident. She learned that her apartment-mate had been puzzled by the way their relationship had changed. Moreover, she was glad to discuss the situation and clear herself of any blame. She too had been missing money, and, when they reported it to the housing supervisor, they found out that others had reported similar thefts. An investigation concluded that the guilty person was a cleaning person, who was promptly discharged. This incident provides several insights regarding reality testing: (1) untested and unchallenged beliefs about another person can damage relationships and cause unhappiness, (2) people are often reluctant to find the relevant information; and, (3) fear of getting at the truth will keep a person increasingly out-of-touch with reality.

Seeing is Believing. Or is it?

Even though we may see or experience the same events, people will have different perceptions, opinions, and feelings. Viewing a video of a police officer shooting a suspicious suspect or being an eye-witness to a crime or an argument is often not sufficient to establish undeniable "facts."

If you have visited St. Louis, Missouri, you have likely seen the Gateway Arch on the Mississippi River. Is the arch taller or is it wider? Since vertical lines look larger than horizontal lines, it looks taller even though the height equals the width.

Look at these two tables in an illustration borrowed from Roger Shepard.[104] If you are like most people, you see that the left table looks longer and narrower than the right table. Take the time to measure with a ruler the dimensions of the two tables. In actuality, the two tables are identical in their dimensions! Magicians, con-artists and politicians use human misperceptions to their advantage and to our loss.

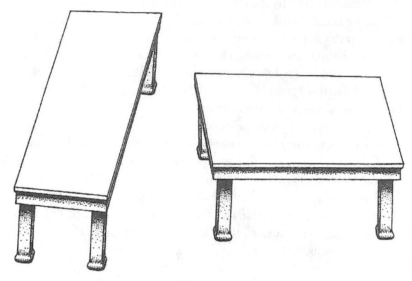

Figure 6.1

In 2017, the Midwest Innocence Project and the Paul E. Wilson Defender Project at the University of Kansas worked to gain the release of a wrongfully convicted man from prison after having served seventeen years of a nineteen-year sentence. Richard Jones had been convicted for aggravated robbery stemming from a 1999 purse-snatching at a Walmart parking lot.

Based on only an eyewitness's testimony, Jones was convicted. Although the accused continually proclaimed his innocence and had a verified alibi, and there was no DNA, fingerprints or any physical evidence, he was convicted based upon the eyewitnesses' accounts.

The subject was identified from a lineup that contained men vastly different from the suspect in appearance. In prison, the other inmates talked about another prisoner who looked just like him. After a two-year endeavor, the Innocence Project found the man who looked like Jones. The following photographs show the resemblance. After looking at the original line-up and the new photos, the judge ruled that no juror would have found the accused guilty in light of the new evidence.[105]

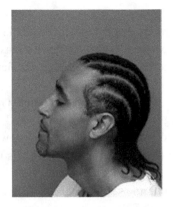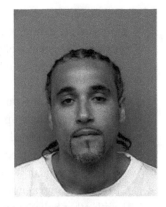

Suspect A, Richard Jones

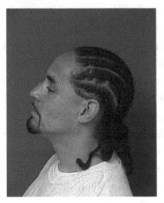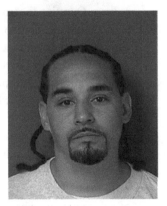

Suspect B, Ricky Amos

In recent years, platforms such as Twitter, Facebook, and Google have allowed distribution of information that is polarizing, misleading or even false. Foreign-sponsored targeted misinformation campaigns have attacked our democratic system and are capable of doing even greater damage. Computer scientists at the University of Washington have successfully built a program capable of creating believable videos of celebrities or political figures saying things they did not actually say. This technology can erode authenticity and the integrity of what or whom we can trust.[106]

Guide for Reality Testing

Reality testing has been mentioned in Chapter 3. If you want to excel at reality testing, master these guidelines. They can be applied to interpersonal communication as well as all media.

1. **State the belief clearly**. Be as specific as possible in your own mind. Are there qualifiers or circumstances that make the situation unique? Where are you on a continuum from certain to possible? Is the belief

closer to definite or to possible?

2. **Examine the evidence that supports this belief**. How credible and reliable is the source of your data? Does the *source* have a bias? Is there clear verification? Make certain you have valid, verifiable, unbiased information.

3. **'Think outside the box" when interpreting the evidence.** Good investigators depend upon seeing the evidence in a new light. Look beyond categories labels and stereotypes. Abandon expectations when weighing evidence. Expanding your view of the world in this way will deepen contact with reality.

4. **Check for congruency**. Try to determine how consistent the belief is with other beliefs known to be valid. Recognize the biases of news resources you consult, check facts, and consult multiple reports. Question the truth of urban myths and local, national, and international gossip. With political statements, or news, it is possible to consult fact-checking websites. See the list in the Appendix A. Look for reliable unbiased news sources. A list of news sources holding solid reputations for factual unbiased news is included in Appendix B. These lists are in no way intended to be comprehensive lists but the entries can serve as beginning resources for those interested in tracking down the facts. Add your own favorite trustworthy news sources and fact checkers as you verify their reliability for yourself.

5. **Support science and the scientific method of inquiry**. The discipline of science is one where the facts, once they are peer-reviewed and published in scientific journals are subject to tests of validation and repetition. It is only then that results of scientific inquiry are accepted as factual. We must respect and support the findings of the scientific community over claims that have not been tested or that fail to be substantiated by scientific inquiry. We must demand that those who make claims cite reputable confirmation, support, and rely on sound logic to reach their conclusions. We have observed the difficulties that arose over unsubstantiated claims regarding topics of climate change, carbon emissions, vaccine protections and public health preparation for a global pandemic.

Systematic application of these rules will help you align beliefs with reality.

Trust and Risk

Trust is a commonly used term in our society. Researchers have long subjected the topic to sustained research. We rely heavily upon our late colleague, Kim Giffin, who invested over forty years to the study of interpersonal trust. Giffin defined trust as: **the reliance of one person on another in a risk-taking situation in order to achieve an uncertain objective**.[107] Let's apply this definition to a sales situation. You are interested in purchasing an automobile. You are placed in a risky situation: paying too much, being deceived about the salient features of the car, etc. Your perception of the salesperson greatly influences your communication behaviors. The uncertain outcome is whether you will buy a car at a price agreed upon by the two of you. Each of you responds to the feedback of the other, nonverbally as well as verbally. Both of you may be less than candid as you seek the lowest price, and the salesperson seeks the highest margin of profit. Negotiation, persuasion, and even haggling may result.

Acceptable risk is determined by comparing what you have to gain with what you have to lose (exchange a wonderful new car for my savings or going into debt for a lemon). Trust is said to be directly correlated with the amount of risk involved. "That car salesman better be trustworthy if I'm going into debt for the car, he/she is selling". The greater the risk, the greater the need for trust. When an Army platoon leader orders his men to jump out of their foxholes and to charge toward the enemy, great physical risk is involved. Therefore, when the men obey, they have placed high trust in their leader. Less apparent, but no less real, is the psychological risk we take when communicating with others. When a student makes a statement in class, there is a risk of negative feedback from the instructor and fellow class members. When you introduce yourself to a stranger you have decided that the potential outcome is greater than the risk of being turned down or disappointed.

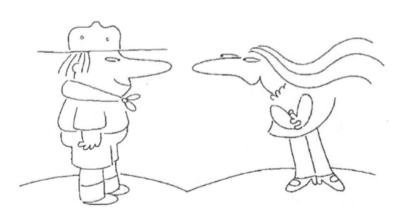

"Well, you certainly don't <u>look</u> trustworthy."

Characteristics Influencing Trust

What do we consider or perceive in another person that makes you believe what he/she tells you? Social scientists are primarily concerned with what you see in a person that gives him/her "source credibility." Three factors appear to be the primary characteristics that others perceive and consider as they decide the degree to which a person can be trusted:

1. Expertness. In all studies of perceived personal characteristics influencing credibility or trust, this factor has been significant. This concept involves perceiving people as experts if they possess knowledge, intelligence, experience, education, training, logic and excellence in judgment. They have specialized knowledge in a special field, such as MDs.
2. Reliability. This factor includes perceptions of honesty, sincerity, goodness, morality, kindness, dependability and patience.
3. Dynamism. The concept of dynamism involves perceived strength, swiftness, aggressiveness, boldness, decisiveness and perceptions of the person as energetic, frank, open, colorful and extroverted.

THE IMPORTANCE OF TRUST

While we have cited the problems and risks in trust, the case is strong for the value of trust and authenticity within our lives and society. Steven R. Covey wrote a book whose title expresses his thesis: *The Speed of Trust, The One Thing That Changes Everything.*[108] Covey believes that trust is the single most important factor that will determine the success or failure of any organization in the 21st century. Efficiency increases when people truly trust one another.

In the book *Extreme Trust*, Don Peppers and Martha Rogers advance the importance of trust in this age of the web, smartphone, and social networks, when every action an organization takes can be exposed and critiqued in real time.[109] Aimed at businesses, the book coins the term "trustability" as a form of "extreme trust." Pepper and Rogers suggest that we think of trust as "a combination of good intentions and competence;" being trustworthy requires "doing the right thing; and doing things right." Good intentions and competency are demonstrated by transparency, sharing data and ideas, utilizing empathy, and reliance on valid information. They conclude, "Very soon, for competitive reasons, all business, old and new, will begin to respond to the increase in demand for "trustability" by taking actions that are more worthy of trust from the beginning – that is, actions that are more transparently honest, less self-interested, more competently executed, less controlling, and more responsible to others' input." Communication will then be healthy for the company as well as the customer.

CAN WE AFFORD TO TRUST?

While distrust protects us, unwarranted distrust limits the fullness of our lives and interactions. This chapter has discussed the dangers associated with misplaced trust, but what case can be made for trusting others? There are at least three reasons for adopting an ethic that increases one's trust of others:

1. Increased trust of others tends to elicit their trust of you. You establish a better climate for cooperative action. In the business world, such cooperation helps you do your job with less tension and fewer interpersonal problems. You can afford to relax and enjoy the company and friendship of co-workers and associates.

2. Increasing your trust of others can improve your own self-image. In many cases, opening up yourself to others will provide an avenue for positive feedback in return, thus validating your desired image of yourself. Also, achieving such feedback, even if negative, can be beneficial and constructive in that you are led to see things in yourself that need improving. In addition, you may obtain helpful suggestions on how such improvement can be made. Usually, along with such constructive suggestions, you also receive from others encouragement to try to change, and stimulation to make the effort because of the potential they see in you.

3. Finally, trusting others increases our chances for psychological health. Being distrustful, defensive, anxious, scared, closed to others, or avoiding interactions all tend to increase your worries and neuroses.

The person who competently identifies trustworthy others will find a source of personal growth and self-development. This person can act with confidence, meeting difficulties and disagreements with poise, laughing and thoroughly enjoying the good things that life has to offer.

WHEN CAN WE TRUST? DEALING WITH RISK AND UNCERTAINTY

In the search for authenticity in society, you must think for yourself and take responsibility for your decisions and your actions. You must improve your competence in dealing with risk and uncertainty. Hopefully, these suggestions will help:

- Circumstances lay the groundwork for whether to trust or not. For many common situations like selling or buying property, repairing a house, or obtaining legal assistance, common practice provides guidelines and safeguards. In strictly social situations, the risks are different and the rigor of your defense mechanisms tends to be lower. Trust until something suggests you withhold further communication.

- Assess your degree of risk through the probability of loss versus gain. In any given situation, assess the likelihood that you will gain your objective. Does this person have expertise on the subject; have they shown reliability in your past dealings? Are they honest and are their motives consistent with your own?

- Trust your intuition. Your subconscious is reading many messages that either make you confident or provoke your stress level. For example, a financial planner may have interests that conflict with yours. Check out any questions that come to mind, seeking validation.
- Verify, verify, verify. Fortunately, technology can give us access to information instantly. In medicine, the discipline of *Evidence-based Medicine* (EBM) has been introduced. Before making a formal diagnosis or judgment, a doctor is encouraged to examine the actual data for epidemiological studies and quantified research. Thus, the doctor's judgment will not be based solely on his/her perspective and experience, but on the best available prior evidence as well.[110] If you want to be trustworthy, you must be able to evaluate information for its objectivity and accuracy before you pass it on.
- Learn to make smart, confident decisions in matters of uncertainty. Everyone must be able to think for themselves. In this world of uncertainty and risk, we need sufficient knowledge of human psychology, an understanding of statistical probability, and the courage to take reasonable risks.

Gerd Gigerenzer, (the Director of the Max Planck Institute for Human Development in Berlin, Germany), has written a timely, insightful book on this topic, *Risk Savvy – How to Make Good Decisions*.[111] After giving a number of examples of how we often badly analyze daily problems and arrive at erroneous solutions, he concludes with sound advice to invest in people. People tend to focus on themselves when stressed. However, a recent Harvard study shows that helping others can significantly decrease the negative effects of stress on the body due to the protective anti-stress effects of the hormone oxytocin. Another study affirmed these findings by showing that people who help others tend to live longer.

As John Adams, the second American president, said in 1765, "Liberty cannot be preserved without a general knowledge among the people." This vision lays the groundwork for participative democracy. Adams' words still ring true for our technological society. Critical thinking requires knowledge and valid information. To keep trust running we need courage, the courage to make our own decisions, take responsibility, and be active participants.[112]

In our world of uncertainty and risk, we have options for the kind of society we will promote. Despite the risks, promote trust in yourself, your close associates, and society in general. Consider who you trust automatically and why (your doctor, mechanic, the people who place labels on canned goods.) Apply similar criteria to unfamiliar parties. Expand your circle of trusted individuals intentionally by considering the aspects of trustworthiness discussed in this chapter.

One of the best ways to incorporate the information from this chapter into your life is to take responsibility for what you say. Distinguish when you are reporting facts or merely stating an opinion. Avoid misleading others into believing that your opinion is demonstrated fact. Empowerment requires truth.

Empowered people trust their own judgements and act to embody the values of fairness, kindness, and self-worth. Strive to use rational/logical thinking to reach conclusions based on factual information. In our personal lives, we screen individuals with whom we interact to decide whether we trust what they tell us and whether to trust them with our personal information, feelings, physical and emotional health, and livelihoods. Everyone can relate the consequences in their own lives of trusting the untrustworthy. When we don't trust people interpersonally, we distance ourselves from them for our own welfare.

A similar process of using rational thinking based on factual information occurs as we make social and political decisions. We need to listen to others with a variety of viewpoints and interpretations to refine our own perspectives, whether that refinement involves agreement on a decision or further discussion of the topics of disagreement. Individuals who cling to an opinion without a logical rationale are not empowered. Skepticism, critical thinking, confirmation of truth, and validation of evidence are required for an empowered life.

The authors recommend recognizing the biases of news resources you consult, checking facts, and consulting multiple reports. Question the truth of urban myths and local, national, and international gossip. With political statements, or news, it is possible to consult fact-checking websites (see the list in the Appendix). A list of news sources that have a solid reputation for unbiased news is included in the Appendix. The bottom line is that empowered people identify the facts and reach their own conclusions regarding the significance of those facts

We began this chapter with an example of deception that resulted in financial loss for Patricia C. We end this chapter with the continuing story of 11-year-old Charlotte McCourt of South Orange, New Jersey, who says truth, trust and honesty are her core values. She cites the Girl Scout Code, "I will do my best to be honest." When the time came for the annual sale of Girl Scout Cookies, she decided to be as honest as possible and tell her customers the whole truth.

She wrote in an internet letter, "The Girl Scout Organization can sometimes use false advertisement." She then proceeded to give each flavor of cookie a rating of 1 to 10: accompanied by a brief critique (at the low end was "Toffeetastic", flavorless as dirt, while "Thin Mints" and "Samoas" received positive reviews She was hoping to sell 300 boxes that year. However, her honesty paid great dividends as she sold 23,219 boxes on 3,551 orders. A CBS reporter, Steve Hartman, said, "Apparently, honesty has become such an aberration, the truth so sadly missed, that when all of these people read Charlotte's letter, they felt compelled to support her...So, America, there is hope that even in a world of *fake news* and *alternative facts*, honesty can and will prevail."[113]

Usually, we expect others to respond openly to what we say. Talk to your trusted friends about openness. Do you almost always respond openly? What might cause you and your friends to be more circumspect than usual in responses? List the people you consider your closest friends. Consider each name and decide if you trust that individual with your personal information. Why or why not? Are there topics you only discuss with male friends? Female friends?

SECTION III – SECOND KEY: EMPATHY

Chapter 7 - Empathy and Personal Health

On January 20, 2008, former U. S. president Barack Obama was invited to address the congregation at the Ebenezer Baptist Church in Atlanta, Georgia. In his address he stated: "The biggest deficit that we have in our society and in the world right now is an empathy deficit. We are in great need of people able to stand in somebody else's shoes and see the world through their eyes."[114] Not only is empathy essential to the health of individuals and to relationships, but it can solve many of our current societal problems. In the years since Obama cited the "empathy deficit" problem in our society, the deficit has only grown greater.

The Importance of Empathy

Researchers have noted, "So much evidence has been accumulated that it is now beyond doubt that being connected and feeling so are beneficial to physical, mental, and social well-being, the three pillars of health defined by the constitution of the World Health Organization."[115]

Empathy is the act of understanding thoughts and feelings of another individual and responding in a way that meets the needs of both communicators. To empathize means to "feel with" another individual. It is different from sympathy, in that sympathy maintains one's own perspective while seeking to console another. Empathy, on the other hand, steps into another individual's awareness or emotional state long enough to understand that person. Empathy connects human beings by allowing one to feel and share the emotions of another. Empathy may very well be the major behavior that most defines us as human. What seems to have begun as an instinctual survival tool has evolved into a sophisticated way of building bonds with others, providing a foundation and the means for expressions of affection, and, ultimately, the ability to understand and get along with individuals vastly different from ourselves.

The process of empathy involves two or more people. True empathy occurs when an individual accurately understands the thoughts and feelings of another individual. The "empathic self," must at different times be able to experience the role of either the sender or receiver of empathy in a healthy manner.

True empathy is an ultimate affirmation of an individual. Empathy has physical and emotional benefits for both the receiver and for the individual who expresses empathy (frequently referred to as the empath or empathizer). Empathy provides a cornerstone for social connection, that element most people consider crucial to a fulfilling life. As reported in *Psychology Today*:

> . . . lack of social connection is a greater detriment to health than obesity, smoking and high blood pressure. On the flip side,

strong social connection leads to a 50 percent increased chance of longevity. Social connection strengthens our immune system. Research by Steve Cole shows that genes impacted by social connection also code for immune function and inflammation, which helps us recover from disease faster, and may even lengthen our life. People who feel more connected to others have lower rates of anxiety and depression. . . . Social connectedness therefore generates a positive feedback loop of social, emotional and physical well-being.[116]

A post 2020 pandemic poll from the Impact Genome Project and the Associated Press—NORC Center for Public Affairs Research—found 18 percent of Americans have one person or no one to help with personal problems such as a ride to the airport or help when ill, and 28 percent say they have only one person or no one to help with work-related problems like writing a resume. African-Americans and Hispanics report this lack of support more often than Caucasians.

ESSENTIAL NEEDS MET BY EMPATHY

Empathic messages meet essential needs in your life.[117] At the most basic level **survival needs** are met when you feel the fears of others, which in turn alerts you to present or potential dangers in your own lives. Certain aspects of empathy seem to be innate.[118] "From an evolutionary point of view, empathy has important survival value assisting individuals in gathering and hunting for food, detecting predators, courtship, and ensuring reproductive success."[119] Innate empathic responses begin in human beings much as they do in other animal life, except that in the human species the effect of empathy exceeds the contributions it makes to other species. In humans, empathic responses affect psychological well-being, social skills and ultimately the achievement of higher levels identified in psychologist Abraham Maslow's hierarchy of needs.[120] In other words, empathy assists not only in meeting basic needs but in securing safety, building community, securing love, developing self-esteem, and meeting potential.

Empathy serves as a **means for relating to others** by providing a basis for sharing commonalities and understanding differences of others. It provides a foundation for developing and maintaining our most meaningful relationships of our lives as well as a way to understand and value those who are most different. As we assume the perspectives of others, we begin to communicate in terms they'll understand, whether we need to express regard or make persuasive arguments from perspectives vastly different from our own.

Empathy can serve as **a source of moral principles**. When we empathize with others, we discover the potential harms of certain acts, the value of fairness, and the importance of providing a fair protection to people, and you recognize a need for moral/ethical codes to establish limits for acceptable behavior. Multiple researchers have connected empathy to helping behaviors and to reducing aggressive behaviors of adults and children, including reducing sexual assaults and domestic violence.

Empathy contributes to the development of individuals as they become a part of society. Individuals learn culturally accepted behaviors and learn to empathize from role models. Infants empathize by mimicking facial expressions, gestures, and emotions of adults with whom they interact. As they become older, children seek through their role-play to understand the nuances of adult life. They pretend to comfort baby dolls and teddy bears. They learn appropriate cultural behaviors and behavioral rules. They practice imagined scenarios and anticipate situations, emergencies, and try on roles and relationships such as "Let's play house," "Let's have a tea party," or "Let's play war." Individuals who do not learn to assume another's perspective cannot learn to empathize. The inability to empathize is associated with states of greater self-absorption such as autism, schizophrenia, narcissism, and depression. A deficiency in ability to empathize interferes with an individual's ability to function effectively and is associated with bullying, violent crime, abusive parenting, spousal battering, and sexual offending. Convicted prisoners have been shown to be limited in their capacity to empathize.

Empathy also serves as a source of self-concept and of self-expansion. As you share yourself and your emotions with others, you reflect on yourself and discover interests, inclinations and values that you may not have recognized on your own. As you empathize with others, you experience emotions vicariously and broaden your own set of experiences, testing your decisions, values, and choices. Marshall Rosenberg supports this assertion by pointing out that "Our ability to offer empathy can allow us to stay vulnerable, defuse potential violence, help us hear the word "no" without taking it as a rejection, revive lifeless conversation, and even hear the feelings and needs expressed through silence.

The Nature of Empathy

Empathy is self-perpetuating. You learn it from those who model it by empathizing with you. It is also reciprocal. The more you provide it to others, the more they provide it to you. The effect reaches beyond a single relationship, for the more an individual experiences true empathy, the more likely he or she is to provide it to others in general. Three different levels of empathy have been identified that meet different needs of communicators. Each occurs in different parts of the brain and, because each involves greater emotional involvement than the other, may be seen as progressively more highly evolved.

1. The first and most basic level is referred to as cognitive empathy. This simply refers to the ability of an individual to identify what another person may be feeling. Empathizing in this way allows individuals to understand "where you're coming from," summarizing meanings and feelings and confirming intellectual understandings, and/or emotions. It is cognitive

empathy that enables a salesman to present a product in a fashion that incites personal interest on the part of a potential buyer or allows a boss to understand the need of an employee to take a day off for personal reasons.

2. The next level of empathy would be **social empathy**, sensing in oneself what another individual is feeling. "I understand your feelings because I, too, have felt this way before." The empath's awareness of self continues to be strong and tends to center on "what I would feel if I were in the other's situation," or "I'm happy that you're happy." The empathizer maintains his or her own ego state.

3. The third level, **true empathy,** demonstrates understanding of perspective, circumstances and emotions. Carl Rogers and other psychologists argue that true empathy goes beyond the first two levels to feel the emotions of another (moving from "I know that you are hurting" and "I hurt because you are hurting" to "I feel your hurt.") True empathy involves an active decision and an investment of oneself and occurs as rare moments of deep connection. True empathy goes beyond intellectual understanding to physical experience and the situating of one's self into the mindset, pertinent history, and present circumstances of another.

EMPATHY BEGINS AS AN INNATE PROCESS THAT CAN ALSO BE TAUGHT

The empathy a child experiences from parents or guardians contributes to the entire being that will develop; "parental empathy fosters positive social response patterns and facilitates the development of adaptive behavior in children." The absence of empathy devastates a child's developing psyche even more than its presence strengthens it.[121] It is worth noting that this expanded role of empathy in humankind also creates an expanded need and application of empathy in the species. The empathetic process can be a natural and automatic response to the emotions of another individual or it can be a more highly developed and controllable reasoned response. Empathy skills in humans can be developed, taught and learned.[122]

Appropriate empathetic responses include the actions performed or words said on the part of the listener to alleviate distress of the discloser. Unfortunately, certain people respond to empathy to alleviate their own feelings of discomfort. If they do not trust their own capabilities, or do not know how to "help," they may, out of frustration, develop defensive, unresponsive, or even aggressive responses. Examples could include the parent who, out of frustration, shakes a crying infant, the children who call a crying child "a crybaby" rather than addressing his/her source of anxiety, the individual who blames another for being victimized, the individual who responds to displays of emotion coldly, or the individual who pretends not to recognize another's emotional distress because he or she is embarrassed by emotional weakness.

At times, a discloser is merely asking to be heard and understood. No advice or solution is being sought. S/he merely needs someone to validate feelings and provide support. Verbal or nonverbal expression of understanding and unconditional regard is all that is needed. In other circumstances, providing emotional support for a course of action or decision is appropriate. At other times, a physical response such as offering a hug, or even just being present but silent are in order. Finally, an offer of assistance or appropriate gift might be an appropriate response (watching children for a stressed parent, bringing groceries to a shut-in neighbor, or giving a stuffed toy to a traumatized child).

Ideally, the appropriateness of an empathetic response is based on the needs of the individual experiencing the emotion rather than the needs of the empath. You sometimes need to remind yourselves that you can meet the needs of others. Everyone is capable of envisioning a solution and imagining a variety of possible actions that might bring about that solution and ultimately figuring out what, if any, part you can play in that solution. Your last action as empathizers is to ask yourselves to answer the following set of questions specifically: "What does my communication partner need, right now from me? Am I prepared to meet that need? And how can I best meet that need?" The necessity of this step of appropriate empathetic response is reinforced by research that points out that the individuals who are most likely to harm a crying child are those most frustrated by their inability to alleviate its distress.

Unconditional positive regard was identified as an essential aspect of empathy by Carl Rogers. He envisioned a day when genuine empathy permeates society, an ideal situation in which parents raise children to be empathetic by guiding developing behaviors without judging the child. According to Rogers, ideal parenting includes actions on the part of the parent that allow a child to acknowledge the disapproval of impulses while simultaneously registering or feeling loved by parents. This concept, referred to as "unconditional love" or "unconditional positive regard," has proven to be important for adults as well as for children. Parental empathy is an essential component necessary for children to develop strong regard for themselves and emotional health.

Messages of unconditional regard can be achieved through such simple acts as referring to another's actions ("You left your socks on the floor") rather than passing judgments ("You are a slob!") It is much easier and less harsh on the ego to change an action (picking up socks) than changing one's core self (from a slob to a neatnik). Another way of offering criticism recommended by psychologists that would affirm unconditional regard would be to offer criticisms sandwiched between positive remarks or affirmations. Psychologists warn that when you employ this so called "sandwich" method, the word "but" should be avoided.

DEVELOPING EMPATHY THROUGH MINDFULNESS

Signs of empathy can be observed in human infants. When one cries another becomes distressed. Fortunate are the children born into environments that further nurture empathetic development. Adults who lack the emotional foundation, intellectual knowledge, and skills necessary to empathetically respond to others require basic training. In pursuing this course, these people must acquire essential empathetic skills through small intentional steps in which they consider their actions and ramifications, and refine those actions until they are capable of responding to others and situations as though they are perfectly prepared. Those of you seeking to improve your empathic skills must rely on whatever appropriate abilities you have and seek out environments and experiences that will allow you to develop the empathetic skills you need for the rich and rewarding interpersonal experiences you crave. Usually this means interrupting unhelpful automatic responses and consciously choosing new more helpful responses.

One contemporary term used for this process is MINDFULNESS. Jon Kabat-Zinn created the Stress Reduction Clinic and the Center for Mindfulness Medicine, Health Care, and Society at the University of Massachusetts Medical School. He integrated centuries-old Buddhist and Zen practices with scientific findings into a non-religious program known as Mindfulness-based stress reduction (MBSR), which is offered by medical centers, hospitals, and health maintenance organizations. Kabat-Zinn defines mindfulness as "moment-to-moment, non-judgmental awareness."[123] It allows you to be fully present, aware of where you are and what you're doing without being overly responsive or overwhelmed by the world around you. As mindful individuals, you are aware of your circumstances at all times and make conscious choices regarding your thoughts and actions. At any point, a mindful person may choose between three options: 1) progress in an old or habitual way, 2) behave in a new way, or 3) do nothing at all.[124]

Mindfulness allows individuals to be aware of their surroundings, their own physical responses, to what is happening at any given time, to enter fully into an activity, to observe without judgment, and to make choices that affect their physical, intellectual and emotional well-being. Mindfulness has been traditionally developed through yoga and meditation, but more recently journal writing and other methods have been associated with its development. Research indicates that mindfulness brings about "a variety of positive psychological effects, including increased subjective well-being, reduced psychological symptoms and emotional reactivity, and improved behavioral regulation."[125] It is frequently used to manage stress, anxiety and spontaneous unwanted emotional outbursts. It has been linked to increased thickness in the cortex and sensory processing.[126] Mindfulness has been linked to positive physical health: pain management and greater positive results in treatment of cancer, heart disease and depression. It has most recently been found useful in lowering blood sugar levels among overweight women, reductions of stress and signs of aging, and increased feelings of well-being among all women.[127] Mindfulness is especially helpful in improving empathetic communicator skills.

When you wish to achieve empathy, resist evaluating the other person's behavior. If you evaluate them as right or wrong, you will be blinded to the message. Focus on truly understanding them without judging them. Take the empathy exam that can be found on the Greater Good website. https://greatergood.berkeley.edu/quizzes/takequiz/empathy

If the task of developing one's own empathetic skills seems too big a task to undertake on one's own, mental health professionals can provide the honest feedback and guidance necessary for the difficult but highly rewarding endeavor of replacing unhealthy habits with healthful alternatives.

Neurologists have proven that intelligence can improve by learning from mistakes and taking corrective actions. The more the subject believes in improvement, the larger the amplitude of a brain signal "that reflects a conscious allocation of attention to errors. And the larger that neural signal, the better the consequent performance."[128] We now have proof that intelligence isn't a preset thing that is incapable of change. Our brains never stop growing new connections, and keeps strengthening with exercise and use. We can make the shift from a reactive brain to a reflexive one as we shift our habits from the mindless toward the mindful.[129]

Problems Stemming from an Absence of Empathy

Most citizens of the world want basically the same things from their society: sufficient prosperity, an educated populace, good health, a responsive governance system that is neither corrupt nor restrictive of freedom, a sustainable natural environment, and a safe, hospitable social environment. Unfortunately, vast portions of the world live without even the most basic of these essentials. The world too often seems to be divided by race, culture, religion, political boundaries, and other innumerable "us" versus "them" divisions. Wars are raging between countries and within countries.

Tribalism

Tribalism has had a long history in human evolution. Originating in our survival instinct, tribalism became crucial in the development of social networks to promote collective protection, safety and the benefits of communal cooperation. Tribalism took on more negative characteristics when groups started to perceive themselves as unique and more special than other groups. Distinctions were made between "us" and "them." Our tribe members were seen in a positive light, promoting connectedness and positive regard, while other tribes and newcomers were seen for their differences such as skin color, size, other appearance factors, and communication styles. Differences were emphasized rather than similarities and became in some cases the basis for anger, jealousy, and rejection. In the most extreme cases, the outsider was seen as less than human and unworthy of support and friendship.

The multiracial, multicultural mix that is the United States today provides a Petri dish of tribal affiliations. Ethnic, racial, geographic, and political groups—among many—can unite but often divide the population.

Tribalism is seen in the way we portray our enemies. In times of war, tribal feelings are exacerbated to the point that we dehumanize our enemies to make it easier to hate and kill them without feelings of empathy or conscience. We are not killing human beings but rather Nazis, Communists, terrorists, the Vietcong, or ISIS. The reality is, the more we fall into tribal attitudes, the more our lives are consumed with hatred. Our survival instincts take over, and our hostilities are directed at our enemies. This tribal hatred diminishes not only the humanity of the victims, but also that of the haters. An absence of empathy harms all parties involved.

Psychiatric Disorders

All psychopathic disorders are characterized by "a lack of empathy and remorse, shallow affect, glibness, manipulation and callousness."[130] Researchers found that when a psychopathic individual sees pain in others, the brain areas necessary for feeling empathy or compassion do not become active. In fact, the area of the brain known to be typically involved with pleasure registers a response. In the U.S., while about 1 percent of the population is shown to be psychopathic, 23 percent of prison inmates are believed to be.[131] The psychopathic disorder encapsulates the essence of the lack of empathy, a condition shared with the following.

1. *Antisocial personality disorder* seems to come from a reduced ability to feel other people's emotional states, especially fear and sadness. People with such a disorder may actually be good at cognitively perceiving others' intentions, while disregarding the emotional content. They may learn to role-play empathy, if they want to be perceived as having empathy without feeling compassion at all.[132]

2. *Autistic spectrum disorder* (ASD) is a spectrum of developmental disorder that can have marked neuro-cognitive impairment in its most severe form. Children with severe ASD display a wide range of communication deficits, but most experts believe lack of empathy is part of the problem, though the underlying causes of the deficit remain a controversial topic. Recent findings, currently being replicated, suggest that a dysfunction in the mirror neuron system may disrupt the normal development of self-other connectedness, creating mental deficits.[133]

3. *Narcissistic personality disorder* (NPD) is one of the few psychiatric disorders that is characterized not only by lack of empathy but also by dysfunctional interaction patterns. The symptoms additionally include

belief that one is special and unique, exploitation of others, arrogance, feeling of jealousy, and a preoccupation with unlimited success. The symptoms cause significant distress for all parties in an interaction. Although researchers cannot say with certainty what causes NPD, the negative effects on society have prompted considerable worldwide research.[134]

4. Impaired empathy has long been associated with *schizophrenia* and with violence in the general population. Someone diagnosed with schizophrenia is likely to exhibit isolationist behavior and a lack of motivation. Some are delusional, holding firmly to a particular belief despite the obvious evidence that the belief is untrue. Schizophrenics often display fragmented thinking and disorganized speech marked by disconnected replies to questions, and an absence of focus.[135]

Each of these four disorders should be viewed as occurring on a spectrum, ranging from highly psychopathic individuals to lesser impaired stages ending in normality. While a relatively small percent of the general population has these problems, the negative impact on society is excessive. The large numbers of psychiatric individuals incarcerated or among the homeless population highlights the problem. Most have an absence of much-needed remedial care. These problems seem to exist in varying degrees in all parts of the world and badly needs research on prevention measures."[136]

The Problem of Loneliness

The absence of empathy in one's life, that is, no one to share feelings, attitudes, opinions and a sense of reality, provokes loneliness. In a column in 2020, George Will discussed what he labeled "the least understood public health problem – loneliness. Will then quotes from a book by Senator Ben Sasse of Nebraska:

"Persistent loneliness" reduces longevity more than twice as much as does heavy drinking and more than three times as much as obesity, which often is a consequence of loneliness. Research demonstrates that loneliness is as physically dangerous as smoking 15 cigarettes a day and contributes to cognitive decline, including more rapid advances of Alzheimer's disease.[137]

Sasse, as an answer, calls for "new habits of mind and heart…new practices of neighborliness." "Neighborliness" is based upon a feeling of shared empathy.

The reaction to the 2020 pandemic calling for isolation, fueled the cases of loneliness. Prior to the attack of the coronavirus, The Health Resources and Services Administration conducted a study of and determined that friendships reduce the risk of mortality or developing disease and speeding recovery. The National Institute for Health Care Management reported that $6.7 billion in federal spending is attributable to social isolation among Medicare clients, accounts for a 29 percent risk of coronary heart disease and a 32 percent rise in respiratory and pulmonary deaths.[138] The deadly impact of the COVID-19 on our older population, then, came as no surprise.

Unfortunately, there is a dark side of empathy; the insight that empathy provides can be used to manipulate and harm others. The fuller knowledge of individuals that one has, the more "emotional weapons" are at one's disposal. That arsenal of "emotional weapons" allows people caught up in their own emotional turmoil to intentionally or accidentally catch others in emotional fallout as well. Manipulative significant others, rapists, and child abusers use empathy to identify weaknesses in targets before turning those targets into their victims. Unethical people may prey on desires or vulnerabilities of individuals (to be helpful, to be kind, to be courteous, to be respected, to be loved…) to create situations where the target ignores existing warning signals in favor of some overriding desire or taught expectation.[139]

Not only can you use empathy to draw closer to those with whom you wish to develop relationships, but empathy can raise alarms identifying those who would use it against you and in that way. Empathy's sword is also its shield.

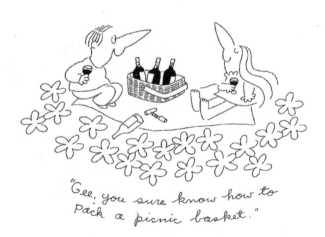

"Gee, you sure know how to pack a picnic basket."

Chapter 8 - Empathy in a Healthy Relationship

Multiple researchers have shown that empathy is important in the development of healthy relationships. The act of having someone empathize with you allows you to feel connected and dispels feelings of loneliness or isolation. Sharing sad news makes it less awful; sharing good news raises the height of celebration; emotional contagion spreads the mood/s of one person to others.

When you empathize with me, my sense of identity is connected to yours. As a result, I feel greater in some way and less alone. I may well, as a result, also start to empathize more with you.[140]

We know that empathy (and improving empathic skills) leads to more positive close relationships, including friendships and romantic relationships. Empathy educators, Charles B. Traux and Robert R. Carkhuff assert that "Empathy is a core component in human relationships and a cornerstone of effective interpersonal skills.[141] Intentional efforts to understand one another build trust and increase relational satisfaction. Through empathy, you establish and maintain friendships.[142] Empathy enhances satisfaction in intimate relationships.[143]

Partners empathizing with each other report deeper connections and understanding of each other. By reducing misunderstandings and increasing understanding of the other's perspective, empathy reduces the number of quarrels and wounded feelings as individuals realize they are fighting over issues, rather than rejecting one another. Empathizing partners are more likely to find ways to help the other and less likely to respond in aggressive acts and bullying.[144] Increased empathy reduces the number of sexual assaults and incidents of domestic violence.[145] It has been found that empathy even increases altruistic behavior. You are more likely to be helpful and generous after an empathic encounter. A willingness to put the other before oneself has the potential for appreciation and reciprocity, all important qualities in a healthy relationship.

Partnering with the right person can make you healthier and extends your life, while linking yourself with the wrong people can make you ill and shorten your life. Louis Cozolino, author of *The Neuroscience of Human Relationships*, emphatically states that, "The correlations between physical health and positive social connectedness are the most consistent and robust findings in the field of psychoneuroimmunology – the study of relationships between mind, body, and physical health."[146] In his summary of the benefits associated with positive social support, Cozolino cites studies that link all of the following to positive social support: general heart health, lower cardiovascular reactions to stress, decreased risk of fatal coronary heart disease, lower blood pressure, lower levels of serum cholesterol, improved immunological functioning, higher levels of natural killer cells, lower urinary cortisol, increased health status and well-being, decreased vulnerability to clinical illness, decreases in symptom display, decreased risk of cancer recurrence, better all-around mental health, decreased depression and anxiety, decreased depression in the elderly, decreased depression during bereavement in men, improved emotional regulation, decreased severity of cognitive decline with age, better sleep, and increased longevity.

Cozolino continues to summarize research that shows, as you would expect, negative relationships are harmful to you as well. In fact, some studies have concluded that negative relationships can have more destructive effects on the body than positive relationships have on healing. Unhappy marriages result in higher levels of stress hormones and lower immunological functions than isolation, especially in women. Critical and hostile others are terrible for your health, correlating with relapses of psychiatric illnesses, hospitalizations, and delayed healing of physical wounds. Abrasive, critical, and hostile close relationships lower immunological functioning and longevity. Chronic stress, conflict and abuse create unhealthy brains and bodies. Being bullied can have serious emotional and behavioral consequences. Victimization results in depression, anxiety, blunted emotions, sleep disturbance, and symptoms of posttraumatic stress disorder. Research demonstrates that biochemical and neurobiological effects of being exposed to predators, negatively impact every level of functioning, from cognition to emotional well-being to longevity.[147]

Empathy impacts families. Some research has demonstrated that improving empathy through family and couples' counseling leads to improved relationships and decreased family problems. Empathy has also been positively associated with family cohesion, parental support, and communicative responsiveness.[148]

It is not an overstatement to say that the quality of the relationships in your life affects the quality of your life. It has been demonstrated that the relationship you have with your doctor, and the empathy expressed in that relationship, affects the accuracy of your diagnosis, your compliance during treatment, and the speed with which you recover. The point here is that as you choose the people who surround you, you are exercising control over your own physical and emotional health and health future.

Understanding the value and process of empathy allows you to gauge the depths of empathy to which you are willing to go. In your shallowest relationships, you might simply mirror another's posture, but in the most important relationships you'll need to give of yourself during the act of empathizing in order to experience fully the benefits of true empathy. As you empathize with others, you not only meet their needs to be understood and your own needs to understand, but you also model the empathic process, convey how you would like to be treated, and anticipate reciprocal treatment. You build atmospheres of trust and deepen your most satisfying relationships.

 To empathize more effectively when listening to a friend, try doing the following:
- Concentrate on understanding both verbal and nonverbal messages.
- Try to feel what the other is feeling.
- Respond appropriately by providing understanding, comfort and support.
- Ask for feedback.
- Ask yourself: Was the effort worthwhile?

Tools for Empathizing

Empathy centers around understanding not only what is said, but the emotions that accompany those words. Mirroring is an interesting phenomenon related to empathy. When you are truly empathizing with individuals you tend to unconsciously mirror their postures, and expressions. When you consciously place yourself in particular postures or facial expressions, you actually feel corresponding emotions. This is a phenomenon you can test for yourself. Conscious physical postures elicit certain emotional responses making it seem as though we can "read minds." Unconscious mirrored movement actually results in emotional understanding as well. A person disclosing important information to you unconsciously picks up on this physical expression of empathy and responds positively.

Emotions are most often conveyed through nonverbal behaviors. Your voice, the looks on your face, and your postures and gestures reveal your emotions even when unintended.

A full emotional vocabulary is essential for expressing emotions and identifying another's emotional state. Robert Plutchik provides a great beginning point by identifying eight basic emotions:

Fear—Anger—Sadness—Joy—Disgust—Trust—Anticipation— Surprise.[149]

Plutchik suggests that any emotion that is not one of the eight basic emotions is a mixture or derivative of them. Some emotions frequently felt but not considered basic by Plutchik include embarrassment, jealousy and guilt. He points out that emotions have degrees of intensity. You should be able to list at least one emotional description that is a toned-down version of the basic eight emotions, and one that is a more intense version. For instance, when you feel mild anger, you might be "annoyed," but when you feel intense anger you could be "furious." As you become adept at describing basic emotions, you'll begin to identify degrees of other emotions as well. Plutchik points out that we name many emotions that are mixtures of two or three emotions, so for example "fear" blended with "surprise" could be referred to as "alarm."[150]

As you seek to understand, ask open-ended questions. These queries convey respect for the distressed individual's unique reactions and responses. The fact that the questioner is sincerely interested, and willing to accept what is said with unconditional regard, is affirming for the other individual.

When providing feedback, use positive words rather than negative words to focus on what the person can still do. Consider pointing out the positive initial goal, "I know how much you wanted to do well on that test." Employing this simple change in language to yourself and to others can actually lift moods, raise optimism levels, and improve interaction climates.

EXPRESSING LOVE, APPRECIATION AND OFFERING COMFORT

Partners who wish to express appreciation, love, or comfort, need to use expressions that are meaningful and with which recipients are comfortable. Have you ever heard someone say, "I'm not appreciated at home," or, "I just don't feel that he or she loves me?" After counseling couples for years, Gary Chapman concluded that we must express love and appreciation in forms that will be understood by our communication partners. His five different expressions of love and regard can also be used to provide comfort. Appropriate expressions are determined by circumstance and the perceptions of the recipient. They might involve touch, words of affirmation, or unsolicited acts of service, quality time, or gifts.[151]

1. **Appropriate and timely touches** involve physical presence and accessibility. They manifest in gestures such as shaking hands, pats on the back, hugs, or holding hands, and in intimate relationships they include kissing, wrapping arms around each other, cuddling, as well as more intimate acts. Using touch to express affinity and appreciation is reliant on whether a partner is receptive to touch. Uninvited use of touch could result in invasion of personal space, uncomfortable exchanges, and even charges of harassment, so it is extremely important to be aware of a partner's appreciation and willingness to experience this expression.

2. **Words of affirmation** involve kind and encouraging words, specific compliments on projects, unsolicited compliments, telling someone the reasons they are appreciated and in love relationships being told "I love you." The power of a "thank you" is amazing. Researchers have determined that expressions of gratitude can predict the quality of a marriage.[152] These words are cherished by individuals whose primary relational language is words of affirmation. For those who prize words of affirmation over

other expressions, the absence of affirmation hurts. Careful forming of criticisms is essential as these individuals can be devastated by criticism. Criticisms are easier to take and feel less like rejections when they include behavior to be changed, interpretation, impact, requested behavior change, positive regard, and willingness to facilitate the change as necessary. For example, "When you arrive late to our production meetings, other team members take it as a sign of disrespect, the meeting is disrupted, and we lose momentum by having to update you. Your creative solutions really help us out. Are there circumstances we should address to make it easier for you to be prompt?"

3. **Unsolicited acts of service** are perceived as unspoken expressions of appreciation, comfort, and love when they are motivated by caring rather than obligation. Expressions can be endless; the individual who, when asked to put some dessert on a plate for a spouse, chooses the prettiest and biggest piece of cake; the father who changes the oil in his daughter's car each time she returns home from college; spouses who take over their loved one's chores when that loved one is overwhelmed at work. Acts at work or at home may be preceded by, "Let me take care of that…" They can relieve us of time pressures and other stressors. At work, this promotes a sense of teamwork and appreciation. The individual who primarily perceives unsolicited acts of service as expressions of love, appreciation, or comfort will feel hurt by laziness, broken commitments or the leaving (or making) of work for them to complete. In times when they need comfort, loving care will allow people to feel safe, cherished, and prepare them to face the world. The mother or wife who complains that "you act like I'm your housekeeper" may actually be complaining that leaving work for her makes her feel unappreciated or unloved. Acts of service provided to someone who is mourning the loss of a loved one may serve to remind him or her that all love is not gone, that s/he is not alone in the world.

4. **Sharing of quality time** may manifest differently in loving relationships and work relationships but is none-the-less an essential expression. It involves undivided attention without distractions. At work, it may manifest in periodic meetings or the willingness to make time for impromptu meetings. At home, family members might turn off phones and televisions to prepare and eat meals together. Parents might schedule alone time with each child. Spouses may set specific "date nights." Whether sitting and talking directly to each other, playing or working, there is an opportunity to focus directly on each other and the problems, celebrations, and updates that keep us involved in each other's lives. Distractions, postponed activities, and failures to listen, send messages that deny love, comfort, and appreciation to those who see these as primary indicators of love or

appreciation. In a subsequent chapter, we will propose regular "healthy communication" sessions.

5. **Giving gifts** as an expression of love, appreciation or comfort is not the same as materialism. There is something special about the thought that goes into a gift; the fact that in the midst of some activity something reminded you of our loved one; that you saw something that will make your loved one smile. There is comfort in the idea that you know them well enough to identify something they will find beautiful, that will make their life easier, or that makes you think of them when you are apart. Gifts send the message that you are prized over whatever was sacrificed to bring the gift to you; this was the message behind the well-known O. Henry story "The Gift of the Magi." While bonuses at work send a message of appreciation, so too does the boss who brings donuts to go with the coffee, a cake for each employee's birthday, or coffee for the break room.

The Role of Empathy in Resolving Conflict

Conflict is a natural, albeit uncomfortable, aspect of any relationship. Empathy can assist you in resolving conflicts. Empathy comes into play in conflict resolution because the first thing that needs to be determined is the problem. Allowing an individual to express the problem in its emotional complexity, and truly listening for the emotions in the situation, can allow parties to feel "heard." Paraphrasing becomes important.

Suppose a couple doesn't have enough money to both renovate the master bathroom and take a vacation to Hawaii. However, that statement may not accurately describe what each of them wants. In this example the husband wants to completely renovate the master bathroom before black mold damages it and he wants a shower large enough to wash away the stresses of the work day. He also wants a spa tub because he knows how much his partner likes to relax in them, and he'd feel guilty giving himself the shower and denying her the tub. The other partner describes her wants: time alone with her husband in a tranquil location without the intrusions that occur at home. They've not been having "us time" lately, and she yearns for the connection that they usually experience, and to give up some of their daily stresses and reconnect.

It's going to take a while for these underlying desires to come out, and they may never surface if the spouses interrupt each other in the telling. Once they empathetically listen to each other, and confirm that what they "understand" is what each person means and feels, then they can look for "win-win" scenarios that meet all essential needs, or at the least, they can consider compromises that meet their most urgent needs. If they identify the overlapping needs that both expressed – connection, affirmation of their love, reduction of stress, doing something nice for each other, and time together—they will ultimately pinpoint their individual prioritized goals: protect the house from black mold, improve bathing facilities, and opportunities to "destress." Then they can work together to find ways to meet all their needs. Instead of a complete bathroom renovation, they check for and repair black mold as a first priority, and put in a new roomy shower. Instead of a spa tub, the husband commits to taking the kids to the park at the same time every week so his wife can relax in the new roomy shower. Instead of going to Hawaii, they choose a resort with similar amenities only a few hours' drive from home, perhaps even during off season so they will be even more isolated and budget conscious. Notice that the solution comes from clearly identifying each person's needs and wants without locking into the solution or win-lose options.

Differences in National Leadership during the 2020 Pandemic

At the beginning of May, 2020, the world responded to the contrasting expressions of empathy by two nations' leader – New Zealand and the United States.

New Zealand is a small country, its total population less than New York City, and is remote with a sealable border, factors that proved to its advantage during the pandemic.

New Zealand's Prime Minister, Jacinda Ardern, was planning to mark the first anniversary of the Christchurch Massacre on March thirteenth with a national memorial event. When the World Health Organization declared a pandemic, the Prime Minister responded immediately and strongly; the event was cancelled; and everyone coming to New Zealand had to self-isolate for fourteen days; a week later, complete lockdown of the country was imposed.

While there was some criticism over the government's action, the overwhelming response was positive, citing clarity of the message and decisiveness of the actions. Unlike countries like the U.S., that declared "war on COVID-19," Ms. Ardern urged people to "Unite against COVID-19" and she referred to the country as "our team of five million."[153]

Professor Michael Baker, from Otago University's Public Health Program in Dunedin, NZ, commented to the BBC, "Jacinda (Ardern) is a brilliant communicator and an empathic leader. What she said made sense and I think people really trusted that. There's been a high level of compliance."[154] He then added that science and leadership have to go together.

The Prime Minister went regularly on Facebook, always smiling and sharing anecdotes from her personal life, but she never underplayed the seriousness of the situation. She repeatedly said she wanted to "check in with everyone" and every decision was made with kindness and decisiveness. She also announced that she, the ministers in her cabinet and public service chief executives would take a 20 percent pay cut for the next six months, to recognize the impact of their fight against the pandemic on all citizens.

The result of these actions was, as of May 15, 2020, NZ had 1500 cases and

96

twenty-one deaths. This amounted to only four deaths per one million people, the lowest number of deaths per capita in the world. By contrast the United States had 1.4 million cases with 84,000 deaths (4,300 deaths per million people). We have repeatedly reported on the leadership in the U.S. during the pandemic. *The Washington Post* declared in the headline of an editorial on April 2, 2020 by Michael Gerson: "We've officially witnessed the total failure of empathy in presidential leadership." Sixteen months later in September 2021, NZ reported a total of only 26 deaths while the US reported over 715,000.

Gerson suggests that "to brag that the television ratings for his afternoon briefings rival those of 'The Bachelor' or 'Monday Night Football' is not mere pettiness. It is clinical solipsism. Exploiting this type of tragedy in the cause of human vanity reveals Trump's spirit to be a vast, trackless wasteland. Trump seems incapable of imagining and reflecting the fears, suffering and grief of his fellow citizens."[155]

Chapter 9 - Empathy in a Diverse Society

Empathy is more than a set of skills. It requires the willingness to step outside yourself and your point of view. You must be able to assume the internal frame of reference of another, and then share back subjective and immediate personal reactions to show your understanding. "I feel what you feel as you feel it." The greater the differences between people, the more difficult empathy is to achieve.

Empathy Issues in the United States

A definition of healthy society as stated in chapter 1 is *a conglomerate of interdependent contributing citizens who create and endow their government with deserved trust and the power necessary to peacefully coordinate and meet the needs of its citizenry, while peacefully co-existing with other societies.* Empathy is necessary to each part of that definition.

The role of empathy in a democracy is to promote understanding between people who differ in many ways but must still work together to promote equitable distribution of resources, opportunities, and privileges within the society. Empathetic societies progress through stages of tolerance, understanding, acceptance, integration, and facilitation to bring problems to successful and peaceful conclusion.

Concerns have arisen over the lack of empathy in America today. David Noise wrote in *Psychology Today*: "the country's political dynamics – the interactions between candidates, the policy proposals being considered, and even the conduct of ordinary citizens – increasingly reflect a complete lack of human empathy, a view toward others that is willfully insensitive, if not outright contemptuous."[156] This lack of empathy has been further demonstrated by voter support for policy proposals that are hostile to immigrants, and a military proposal by one presidential candidate in 2016 to "carpet bomb the Middle East" to the point where "sand can glow in the dark." Both examples show a total lack of concern for the loss of life and suffering of innocent humans.

All categories of diversity –religious, sexual orientation, ethnicity, and gender to name a few– have been played against one another. As Noise points out, our discourse is uncivil to the extent that in "today's America, from our presidential candidates to our blogospheres and major media more often (than not) thrives on outrage, emotion and personal attacks."[157]

All of us are capable of making moral choices. Making the right choice is more difficult for people with compromised empathy circuits, but the choice still must be made. We believe that lack of empathy needs to be viewed as a health problem. For severe cases, a medical setting will be more appropriate for remediation than a prison. Why is it that we resort to punishments, violence and bullying so often in trying to resolve conflict? Punishments have been found to be ineffective ways to modify behaviors: "To punish a man you must injure him: to reform a man you must improve him, and men are not improved by injuries."[158] A Harvard study concluded that in an extremely competitive setting, the winners resisted the temptation to escalate conflicts, while those who relied on punishments to get what they wanted consistently lost.[159] We know that punishment alone does not reform. Understanding the circumstances that bring about a reprehensible crime helps to determine how to make lawful behavior appealing and diminish the factors that promote the behaviors in the first place. Empathy allows us to identify those individuals who cannot be trusted in society, and what must be changed before allowing them back into society.

We have pointed out that a world without empathy is chaotic and uncivilized. Empathy creates bonds of trust, provides insights as to what others are thinking and feeling, and informs the choices and decisions we make.

Problems during the COVID-19 Pandemic

The coronavirus pandemic in 2020 led to sweeping changes and disruptions in nearly every aspect of daily life. With ongoing updates of guidelines and mandates and illness and death counts, people felt overwhelmed with anxieties. Empathizing with others makes both parties feel less lonely and more connected.

The absence of societal empathy in the U.S. created and exaggerated some problems. A small group of people hoarded supplies like toilet paper, even though having these items was not going to protect then against the virus. As a result, even more people began hoarding supplies. A man purchased all of the toilet paper in one town and was arrested for selling rolls at inflated prices in the Wal-Mart parking lot. The hoarders thought nothing of how these actions would affect everyone else – and didn't care.

The absence of empathy is explicit in statements overheard and read on the internet such as "We shouldn't care about a lot of people dying. Everybody is going to die sooner or later anyway." During 2020, doctors, nurses, and service providers were all putting their lives on the line, only to be met with disregard and unnecessary recklessness. The elderly, parents with children, and furloughed workers had to fend for themselves. As the death numbers grew, some Americans continued to crowd beaches and bars, socializing as usual despite the warning from health care officials.

As social distancing and isolation to prevent illness grew, in-person communication choices diminished, but instead of turning inward and focusing solely on self, social media became the way to meaningful connections and actions. Recall that research has shown that caring for others is one of the best ways to fight feelings of isolation. With added time available to many, they connected with friends and relatives through snail mail, emails, Facebook, zoom and phone calls to keep or reestablish connectedness.

Societal Development of Empathy—A Case Study

Community tensions, social and otherwise, can be eased by using an empathy-centered approach to empower the people on both sides of a conflict. A young minister named Lloyd Henderson, in a Wyoming town of about 9,000 people, was concerned about the sharp division between the Mexican-Americans and Anglos in the community. The town was divided physically by railroad tracks with the Mexican Americans (about one fourth of the population) on the south side and Anglos on the north. The Anglos thought everything was fine and said there was no discrimination. The Mexican-Americans, however, felt oppressed and believed the community was unresponsive to their needs. Anger was growing and moving from passive resignation to burning resentment.

The minister secured a modest grant for a program designed to improve communication between the two groups. He selected nine leaders from the community representing a cross-section of groups: Anglo, Mexican Americas, men and women, upper class, middle class, and lower class. These leaders were given intensive training on how to facilitate a group to focus on being genuine and to truly listen to one another. Nine groups were then set up consisting of one of the leaders and eight to fifteen members each. They met once a week for twelve weeks, with an optional weekend meeting. Each group was chosen for maximum diversity. For example, one group had a local judge and a couple of Mexican American youths who feared him.

When the leaders purposefully remained passive and refused to take on traditional leadership functions, the members realized that they had to take responsibility for the functioning of the group. The conversations became both personal and focused on community problems with talk about unemployment and educational concerns. The Anglos admitted that they considered Mexican Americans to be a unified group, while the Mexican-Americans felt an absence of solidarity within their group and believed that their lack of cohesiveness was a barrier to progress.

One of the characteristic discoveries across all the groups was that the attitudes of the participants, no matter their backgrounds or ages, were more similar than they had supposed. When discussing their children or the need for meaningful employment, feelings were the same on both sides of the tracks. Two mothers, one Mexican-American, one Anglo, expressed awe and wonder at how similar they were in their hopes for their children, as well as their feelings about other problems.

Gradual changes began to occur. People who in the usual course of events would never have met, built friendships across cultural and age barriers. The judge expressed a greater understanding of the youths he encountered. Some groups even took action, such as talking to employers about their hiring practices.

After the group sessions ended, the Mexican Americans met as a group, bonded together and wrote a proposal for a grant from the federal government, aimed at reducing school dropouts, providing job training, and taking parents for a visit to the near-by state university to elevate educational aspirations. The proposal was funded, and it proved a morale booster for the whole community. Individuals from both groups became empowered because they were able to realize their strengths through authentic and empathic communication.[160]

A documentary film, *Strangers in Our Town (*www.strangersintownthefilm. com*)*, vividly illustrates what can happen when a community chooses to embrace immigrants. The filmmakers, Steve Lerner and Reuben Aaronson, tell the story of Garden City, Kansas, a conservative town of 14,000, in the late 1970's that gains two large packing plants and an explosion of immigrant laborers and their families. By 2015 the town had grown to 26,000 and 26 languages were spoken in the high school.

The film shows that through thoughtful planning and strong, determined leadership, the town embraced this diversity. Filmmaker Steve Lerner noted, "One thing that's clear to me is that there was a group of people in city government, the law enforcement community, the schools and the religious community that made an explicit decision to make this work in their town." To underscore that perception, the town's emblem became a multicolored yucca plant and the town motto changed to "The world grows here."

Garden City made national news the day following the 2016 presidential election when three men were arrested for planning to bomb an apartment complex that housed more than 100 Somali Muslim immigrants and a mosque. None of the arrested were from Garden City, but members of a Kansas militia knew of the city's inclusive policies and planned to target the immigrants. When the plans were disclosed, Garden City banded together in large numbers to support their immigrant residents. The film demonstrates how acceptance and positive regard can bridge differences.

We all know that it is much harder to hate and hurt people you truly know and understand. You are unlikely to be indifferent to the suffering of a person or persons that you know and identify with. Consider the two extremes of your feelings for other people: disdain, indifference and hatred at one extreme; empathy, compassion and love at the other. You can choose to understand others' points of view and feelings in the workplace, your neighborhoods, your places of worship, and through discussions with family and friends.

Spread the core values of empathy to improve lives, health, meaningful relationships and better decision making. Teach children to be empathetic. When someone makes you feel that you are valued and cared for, you are likely to feel good about yourself, and are more likely to show your care in return. It's a virtuous cycle; keep it going. Because the brain's neural circuitry is malleable, and as such can be rewired and changed, your tendency for empathy and compassion is never fixed, but with thoughtful choices, empathetic behaviors can be increased throughout your life.[161]

Listed below are some of the many ways to rehearse, inform and increase your empathic understanding of other people:

1. Participate in the arts, attend the theatre, see challenging films, read widely, play educational computer games, and allow yourself to feel and absorb various kinds of music.
2. Travel to other countries and communities and absorb other cultures.
3. Start a conversation with someone very different from yourself. Try to get to know them.
4. Take opportunities to share experiences with someone unlike yourself and talk about your reactions and feelings.
5. Encourage and support school programs that teach about empathy and emotions. Dr. Carol Kusche, a psychologist in Seattle, has developed a well-researched curriculum, currently used in Seattle and other U. S. cities as well as in twenty foreign countries.[162]
6. Exercise regularly. Exercise has been linked to greater empathy and needs to be encouraged for everyone.
7. Volunteer for charitable causes. Volunteering is good for your health and for your development of empathy.
8. Meditate and/or practice mindfulness. Recent studies have shown that meditation and the new practices of mindfulness can rewire your brain. One activity is call LKM (loving-kindness meditation). The meditation takes a few minutes a day and focuses on sending loving and compassionate thoughts to family, self and friends, especially those with whom you have tension or a conflict.[163]

Collectively, these small steps can help make you a more caring person and the world a better place.

Technologies exist and are being further refined that allow individuals or nations to impact people with whom they never physically meet. We can now know specific individuals around the globe, are able to talk with (or fight or insult) anyone on earth, and we are able to travel to its most remote locations. The technologies are a gift in providing opportunities for far-away friends, but also increase the possibility of more enemies. We find ourselves interacting with individuals vastly different from ourselves, working together for common goals, helping each other, and resolving conflicts. Like it or not, each of us is now a citizen of the world and the rest of the world's residents are our next-door neighbors.

We've already discussed that researchers have found that kindness is more likely to be met with kindness, empathy is more likely to be met with empathy, and empathy encourages selfless actions. When science and common sense agree, we should heed the conclusions. When empathy is combined with reflective response, humankind benefits. Just as healthy individuals have no need or desire to harm themselves or others, healthy societies develop healthy attitudes toward not only those like themselves but also toward those who are different.

Developing Empathy with People from Other Cultures

Communication style includes verbal and nonverbal cues, as well as their meanings, and the importance we attribute to each. Some cultures are straightforward in their use of language while others are more circular following elaborate rules of etiquette. Sensitivity to what people are "saying without speaking" is extremely important and understanding potential causes of offense is essential. Some cultures value words, while others value silence. Eye contact and spatial boundaries can communicate friendliness or aggression. Raised voices indicate amount of involvement in the discussion for some while it indicates anger in others. What is considered an appropriate degree of assertiveness, and what is considered confrontation differ from culture to culture. In the U.S., we usually encourage people to deal directly with problems as they arise, heading off full-blown conflicts; however, eastern countries view open conflict as embarrassing or demeaning, with differences resolved quietly, perhaps in a written exchange.

Approaches to completing tasks can vary based on access to resources, different judgment of the rewards associated with task completion, different notions of time, and varied ideas about how relationship building and task-oriented work should go together. While all cultures value the productivity of individuals who can work together, some cultures (such as Asian and Hispanic) tend to attach more value to developing relationships at the beginning of a shared project, and more emphasis on task completion toward the end. Cultures such as Europeans and Americans tend to focus immediately on the task at hand and let relationships develop as work on a task progresses. Notice that both ideologies value productivity and relationships; they simply approach their development differently.

Expectations about roles and preferences for the process to be used in decision making are influenced by your culture and include attitudes toward majority rule, consensus, and whether the leader is expected to delegate the responsibility for a decision. While Americans are usually quite comfortable with majority rule, there are cultures who consider it shameful when groups cannot reach consensus.

Attitudes toward disclosure are also something to consider before you begin analyzing the views, experiences, and goals of people from other cultures. What information is easily shared and what subjects are taboo? Questions regarding certain subjects could help in developing empathetic attitudes but may be considered intrusive. It is important to recognize that, regardless of your good intentions, all questions may not be welcome.

Different approaches "to knowing" also vary from society to society. European (and American) cultures value information acquired through cognitive means and hold knowledge gained through scientific method to be more valid than other ways of coming to "know." Some cultures may prefer "affective ways of knowing" such as symbolic imagery and rhythm, while other cultures may emphasize the validity of knowledge gained through intuition.

We must remember that humans' strongest advantage over other species is our ability to work together cooperatively in groups. Reason was developed, in large part, to help resolve problems posed by living in collective groups.

For a healthy society, the use of empathy may mean looking deeper at the experiences of individuals or cultures with whom we don't necessarily identity or agree. Remember that we do not have to endorse an action to understand the circumstances and attitudes that brought it about. Such understanding increases the likelihood of better societal decision making.

Optimism for a More Empathic Future

We recognize that we have painted a grim picture of the current status of empathy in our society. The past few years have offered ample evidence that in this country and others, the governing elite and the massive bureaucracies that support them have no place for dissenters or those with different values and goals. Acceptance of diversity of values, lifestyles, and opinions is at the heart of the democratic process but on many ways, it seems to be no longer flourishing in America.

We believe that the U.S. political reactions of today are often in response to the social changes of the past decade such as the growing number of minorities and the acceptance of homosexuality, bisexuality, transsexuality. The Obama era saw greater equality for women in the marketplace, free health clinics, family planning assistance, alternative schools, and expanding opportunities for a diverse population. These changes created frightened, angry people who yearned for the old status quo. Change is painful.

As we started this book, we articulated the fact that change is the one constant in life. People and society are continually in process. Possibly, by the time you read this book, a shift might have already begun toward a more empathic society. The seeds are being planted every day.

In 2009, Jeremy Rifkin wrote an optimistic book entitled *The Empathic Civilization*. At this time of crisis for our environmental future, Rifkin saw an expansion of consciousness as we move into an "Age of Empathy." He began his book with the most important question facing humanity: "Can we reach global empathy in time to avoid the collapse of civilization and save the Earth?"[164]

Taking a process perspective, Rifkin cited the "human activity" of burning fossil-fuels as a major threat to the climate of Earth and all living creatures. He went on to state:

> Our dawning awareness that the Earth functions like an individual organism requires us to rethink our notions of global risks, vulnerability and security. If every human life, the species as a whole, and life-forms are interwoven with one another and with the geochemistry of the planet in a rich and complex choreography that sustains life itself, then we are all dependent on and responsible for the health of the whole organism.[165]

The solution, according to Rifkin, lies in the classroom where we must teach the need to be energy efficient, and how students must have a deeper sense of interconnectivity and social responsibility. Most importantly, empathic development must help students make emotional connections with people in all parts of the world. He outlined a global empathy curriculum that begins in the first grade and proceeds at each grade level. Tens of thousands have gone through these "Roots of Empathy" programs in eighteen states and Canada, and have documented enormous changes with "a marked reduction in aggression, violence, and other antisocial behavior, a decrease in disciplinary actions, greater cooperation in the classroom, a greater desire to learn, and improvement in critical thinking skills."[166] These same principles can be applied to other tribal behaviors such as in reintegrating the military back into our society. If we have trained soldiers to act without empathy, we have a responsibility to restore those feelings.

Written before President Trump's decision in 2017 to withdraw from the Paris Climate Accord, Rifkin believed the availability of renewable energies will level the international economic "playing field" and prompt a new communications revolution that will in turn broaden empathic sensibility. This new world will be de-centralized and autonomous. If such action falls into place, Rifkin provided the optimistic prediction:

> The new biosphere politics transcends traditional right/left distinctions so characteristic of the geopolitics of the modern market economy and nation-state era. The new divide is generational and contrasts the traditional top-down model of structuring family life, education, commerce, and governance with a younger generation whose thinking is more relational and distributed, whose nature is more collaborative and cosmopolitan, and whose work and social spaces favor open-source commons. For the Internet generation, "quality of life" becomes as important as individual opportunity in fashioning a new dream for the 21st century.[167]

Since America's renewed commitment to support the accord in 2021, there is cause for optimism by the positive actions in other countries. According to *Bloomberg New Energy Finance*, as countries around the world are investing more in renewables, the prices for solar panels, equipment such as photovoltaic cells and wind turbines are dropping, making them more accessible.

Also, *Bloomberg* predicted that in the near future, Germany will get 50 percent of its energy from renewables, and China's investment in solar power will make it less expensive than natural gas. By 2029, solar and wind power will be cheaper than coal in the U.S., Germany and China. By 2038, the world will get 50 percent of its energy from renewables, distributed evenly across hydroelectric, solar and wind power.[168] We have cause for optimism that economic pressures will augment the scientific evidence of climate change, and help bring Rifkin's predictions to fruition.

In his 2018 book *Enlightenment Now*, Harvard cognitive psychologist Stephen Pinker pointed out that our current negativism and pessimism come primarily from a system of psychological biases and mental traps that cause us to accentuate the negative and downplay the affirmative. With the mass media emphasizing the bad news over the good, we fail to notice and acknowledge the widespread improvements in the human condition that are indeed happening globally.[169]

In seventy-five surprising graphs, Pinker shows historically and globally that improvements have been made in life, health, wealth, equality, sustenance, peace, safety, democracy, the environment, knowledge, quality of life, and happiness. He makes a strong case for reason, science, and humanism, the ideals we need to confront our problems and continue our progress.

As an example, we look at Pinker's analysis that underlies his belief that the world environment is improving. The key to dealing with the reality of climate change is to produce the most energy with the least emission of greenhouse gases. The world's economic progress has demanded more energy, yet for the past half century, carbon emissions have been declining. This positive change is due to such factors as replacing coal with gas and greater use of zero-carbon nuclear energy. With the world now focused on the problem, policy and new technology will help us rise to the challenge. On August 9, 2021 the United Nations scientists announced "a code red for humanity." Their report calls climate change unequivocally human-caused.

Pinker was partially wrong in the view that world-wide life expectancy would continue to rise. His data on the U.S. dated back to 2015 was true then. In the past six years, however, a surprising and disquieting trend has come to light. The U.S. life expectancy, unlike the rest of the world, has declined, some in 2016 and more in the four subsequent years. Drug overdoses in 2017, for example, accounted for 70,000 American deaths and suicide another 47,000. Stanford University Behavioral Scientist, Keith Humphreys correlates increased gun ownership with increased suicide rate. He points to the fact that the suicide rate of rural residents (20 per 100,000) has gone up sharply compared to urban Americans (11.1 in 100,000). Nearly 60 percent of rural homes have guns versus less than half of homes in urban areas. As Humphreys states, "Having easily available lethal means is a big risk factor for suicide."[170] The decisions America has made on guns and opioids have taken its toll on American life expectancy. Then came the 2020 pandemic.

The evolving empathetic human brain is capable of adjusting to the demands associated with our changing world. Empathy is essential to every aspect in the definition of a healthy society. We employ societal empathy to improve circumstances for members of our own culture (starting with our home, our neighborhood, our state, our country.) We also employ empathy by learning to identify with individuals from different cultures, so we can improve international circumstances. We can understand people from different cultures by paying attention to communication styles, attitudes toward conflict, approaches to completing tasks; decision-making styles, attitudes toward disclosure, and approaches to knowing. We must hold the media, government and ourselves accountable for recognizing those in need of our empathy, and we must meet the challenges of creating social justice. Our world's future depends on the collective quality of our decisions and the actions we take.

SECTION IV – THIRD KEY: EMPOWERMENT

Chapter 10 - Personal Empowerment

"Politics" is a bad word today. Politicians are held in low regard. In present-day social sciences; politics refers to issues of *Power* and *Control*; how people attempt to gain, possess, share or surrender power and control over others and/or themselves. These same issues of power and control are related to personal empowerment.

The Political Basis for Personal Empowerment

The principles of our U.S. Constitution, especially the Bill of Rights, give us the rights to freedom of thought and speech, and the right to advocate even unpopular points of view. At the time of the drafting of the constitution such personal freedoms and the rights of individual citizens were unique, as was our country's reliance upon democratic decision making and a republican form of government. This emphasis on personal liberty contrasts with the concept of the ideal citizen held in other countries. Prior to the American Revolution, political power resided in the hands of monarchs, dictators, royalty, and the rich. In such societies, the ideal citizen was often the "obedient" person, obedient to the leaders of the state.

In 1787, a small group of prominent political leaders from the thirteen states met to draft and ratify a document designed to operationalize representative republican principles on a national scale to replace the Articles of Confederation. These white, male delegates bargained, negotiated, and brokered to produce the constitutional consensus: balancing power between large and small states; federal versus state jurisdiction; and a sectional agreement over slavery. On the overriding question of sovereignty, they stated that it did not reside with the federal government or with the individual states; it *resides with "the people."* No definition of "the people" was provided.

No one had ever established a country of this scale on such principles. The following decade revealed that the interpretations of the framework for our government were a "work-in-progress." The historical divide came between the "Jeffersonians" who focused on protecting the rights of the individual; and the "Hamiltonians" who believed that strong centralized government was the key to the success of the country. To a large extent, this divide persists between Republicans (or Conservatives) and Democrats (or Liberals) today.[171]

The point is that our founding fathers laid the groundwork for personal empowerment, a value that has endured to the present day, despite serious attacks from all phases of society. The first ten Amendments to the Constitution, instigated by James Madison, serve to guarantee these personal freedoms. We now refer to those ten amendments as the Bill of Rights.

Democracy has protected the rights of individuals by rejecting authoritarian practices. Skeptics resist this assumption arguing that the populous does not have the necessary intelligence to truly govern themselves. Sigmund Freud presented the argument in his writing. Consider Freud's views on groups of people and how they undermine the very premise of democracy:

> A group is extraordinarily credulous and open to influence, it has no critical faculty, and the improbable does not exist for it. . . . Inclined as it itself is to all extremes, a group can only be excited by an excessive stimulus. Anyone who wishes to produce an effect upon it needs no logical adjustment on his arguments, he must paint in the most forcible colors, he must exaggerate, and he must repeat the same thing again and again. It respects force and can only be slightly influenced by kindness, which it regards merely as a form of weakness.
> It wants to be ruled and oppressed, and to fear its masters.
>
> And, finally, groups have never thirsted after truth. They demand illusions and cannot do without them. They constantly give what is unreal precedence over what is real; they are almost as strongly influenced by what is untrue as by what is true. They have an evident tendency not to distinguish between the two. . . . A group is an obedient herd, which could never live without a master. It has such a thirst for obedience that it submits instinctively to anyone who appoints himself as the master.[172]

These perspectives with such low regard for human nature were said to have influenced Hitler and other authoritarian leaders. We hope that Freud underestimated the capacities of people. The founding fathers rejected this low assessment of human potential. Our approach to healthy empowerment is based on the premise that a person can be trustworthy, capable of judging reality, understanding self in context, making constructive choices and acting on those choices. America remains divided on the question.

Oppression and Powerlessness

Minorities in our society have characteristically been denied power by the privileged. Anyone who can be identified as different whether due to gender, ethnicity, handicap or sexuality are made to feel inferior and are kept out of the decision-making process. Whether these groups need jobs, equal pay, civil rights, or educational opportunities, these rights must be wrested away from those in power . . . who will not give them up willingly.

Minorities' struggles for rights have been documented since our country's infancy. The unresolved issue of slavery, avoided by our founding fathers, could only be settled by a devastating Civil War (1861-1865). In our lifetimes, we have witnessed various groups fight for and often receive the personal rights they should have had all along. Many of those battles continue to this day.

Our nation's problems are only a part of the world's problems, problems that will decide our future. Modern feuds divide cultures, ideologies, religions, and nations. The current battle for power and control in the Middle East includes the struggle for Syria, the long-standing dispute between the Palestinians and the Israelis, as well as North versus South Korea. Regretfully, these disputes characteristically resort to warfare for resolution. In tense situations, a pattern can usually be identified: each of the participants holds an identical view, with equal convictions.

People seem to be continuously driven toward greater freedom and control over their own lives. Since the beginning of our species, we can trace the nature and motivation that has promoted this evolution. Carl Rogers advanced a theory that provides an understanding to this human desire for personal empowerment.[173] Rogers noted that all forms of life, from plants, to insects, to mammals, all of life exhibits behavior that "can be counted on to be in the direction of maintaining, enhancing, and reproducing itself."[174] This tendency involves a differentiation of organs and function; it involves enhancement through reproduction, and demonstrates a trend toward self-regulation and away from control by external forces.

Rogers further believed that humans are always motivated, always seeking; and such drives empower the person. All of us strive for power to make choices about our well-being, and receive satisfaction from these driving forces through personal growth and more fulfilling lives.

This theory provides optimism for our future as this motivation toward self-empowerment becomes recognized and rewarded. Empowerment is the opposite of victimization. A victim is in a powerless position and someone of greater power has maliciously, ignorantly or from a lack of awareness or concern caused harm to the person. Victims view themselves as powerless individuals who are "done to." The empowered person, on the other hand, refuses to accept a label as victim. Rather than surrender to powerlessness, the empowered individual employs whatever power he or she has.

Dr. Jen's Rx

For...

Address...

Rx   Date:......................

*If we do not provide the young with good
models that they can believe in, they will
seek and find bad models. The most
pressing need of an unformed personality
is to find appropriate models.*

Refills NA 1 2 3 4 5

Signature...

Power and Empowerment

While power generally assumes controlling others, empowerment emerges as a concept depicting control over self and your capacity to self-regulate. Empowerment involves an understanding of the extent of one's own choices and their consequences while recognizing the centers of power at play. "I am not in control of your actions, but I control my own". Despite other's attempts to coerce and influence factors beyond their control, empowered individuals recognize an internal locus of power; while individuals who believe their actions are a result of others, ("they made me do it"), perceive an external locus of power. Empowered individuals recognize that interpreting a message is subjective. They do not automatically accept the limits placed on them by others, and they most certainly don't place unnecessary limits on themselves. The empowered individual refuses to be defined by stereotype or role.

Empowered people also recognize that interpretations are under their control. So, for example, it may be true that "you wagged your finger in front of my face," but whether I believe it was "just a friendly tease" or "an aggressive warning" is my interpretation, and my best recourse would be to check with you before responding. It may be true that "I am angry at you," (assuming my own power) but you did not "make me angry" (asserting that you have power over me.) Likewise, I may do something to which you respond, but I don't "make you love me" or "make you happy (or unhappy,)" nor do I "make you hit me." It is no one's responsibility to assume the emotional welfare or actions of another adult. Empowerment recognizes that you have responsibility for the choices you make, and the consequences of these choices are your own. If a child is permitted to dominate his/her parents, the child has too much power. Through manipulation and tactics such as crying, the child learns he/she can gain control. If such behaviors are allowed to continue unabated, the child may become a bully. The parents gave up their control voluntarily and allowed themselves to be powerless.

In an alternative scenario, the parents refuse to permit their child's behaviors to control them, and instead maintain their own power to shape the child's maturation toward appropriate goals. As the child matures, the parents foster opportunities for his/her empowerment and self-regulation. The child learns that he/she may ask things of others but doesn't, and shouldn't have control over them.

Empowerment became a popular term in the 1970's as women made the case for equality under the law and the same rights afforded to men. These women learned a lesson that has been important to all minority struggles since. To obtain genuine equality, power and power structures must change either by one group's relinquishing it to another, or by expanding the power base. Other groups in our society have learned to exert their influence to promote such change, as in the more recent movement of LGBTQ proponents to gain rights to marry, and for transgender people to have choice of access to public toilets. The "Black Lives Matter" movement came forward in response to disproportionate police violence against the Black community. Empowerment has become a rallying call to change the power structures, and recognize individuals' greater control over their lives and the choices they make.

Class and Health in the U.S.

Stress, poverty, low socioeconomic status, unhealthy lifestyle, and unpleasant living and working conditions are among the many inherently social variables regarded as causes of ill health.[175] Michael Marmot has stated: "The lower the social position, the higher the risk of heart disease, stroke, lung diseases, diseases of the digestive tract, kidney diseases, HIV-related diseases, tuberculosis, suicide, and other "accidental" and violent deaths."[176] A striking example of the impact of socioeconomic status on health can be observed on the Washington DC metro system. From the deteriorated neighborhoods southeast of downtown to affluent Montgomery County, Maryland, life expectancy for the residents rises by about one and one-half years for each mile traveled. There is a twenty-year gap in life-expectancy between the low-income black people at the beginning of the trip and the wealthy whites at the end of the trip. The direct linkage between power and economic status are too obvious to be discussed. Empowerment is similarly related to standard of living.

As elsewhere in the world, class is the strongest and most consistent predictor of health and longevity in the United States. In the case of coronary heart disease, while there has been an overall decrease in the past sixty-five years, the greatest improvements have been in the upper and middle classes. (Routine preventive care is not part of the impoverished lifestyle, and hospital emergency rooms are often the only option.)[177] Earlier in this book we discussed how Adverse Childhood

Experiences have been linked to risky health behaviors, chronic health conditions, low life potential, and early death.[178] These ACE scores are reflections of the physical and environmental stressors children face, and the Center for Disease Control recognizes that addressing these experiences is a public health issue.

Race is not the reason black people in the U. S. have the highest mortality rates for virtually all diseases and illnesses. Blame must instead be cast on levels of income and education.[179] The social research revealing these facts provides a compelling case for national health care and policy efforts to promote empowerment.

Racism in Health Outcomes during the 2020 Pandemic

In 2020, COVID-19 expanded the divide in the U.S. between those ready to explore the structural racism ingrained in the country and those who were not. The Centers for Disease Control and Prevention published daily data on the racial breakdown of confirmed cases and deaths. However, on one date in 2020, with over 900,000 cases documented, only 36 percent were broken down by race, largely because many states and municipalities were not recording racial data! Senator Elizabeth Warren introduced legislation to compel the publishing of daily data broken down by race. She said "Because of government-sponsored discrimination and systemic racism, communities of color are at the frontlines of this pandemic."[180] The Senate failed to advance the bill.

Even without accurate national data, cities and states that noted race reported much higher mortality rates among black communities. In St. Louis, Missouri, in the first weeks of the pandemic, the only people to die from the virus were from the black community. On April 8, 2020 the coronavirus killed twelve people; they were all black people. At the point when Michigan had 3,000 deaths, African Americans, (who constitute only 14 percent of the state's population) made up 40 percent of the death toll. Early in May the Centers for Disease Control and Prevention released its first breakdown of COVID-19 case data by race, showing that 30 percent of patients whose race was known were black.

Decades of segregation, discriminatory housing policies and poor environmental protections have left many African Americans living in substandard and high-density housing, where social distancing is difficult, and areas of greater air pollution, lead to higher incidents of asthma and other diseases, raising risks for those suffering from COVID-19.

Racial and ethnic minorities at all education levels have reported that they are typically less able than white people to handle financial setbacks. Black and Hispanic-owned small businesses have less access to traditional financial lenders, which makes it difficult or impossible to secure access to the coronavirus relief program. Dr. Lisa Cooper, a Bloomberg Distinguished Professor and Director of the Center for Health Equity at Johns Hopkins University stated:

We need to understand that people's health is not a direct result of their behaviors and actions. People's individual actions and behaviors do play a role in health. But the environments in which they exist and the policies that we put in place that shape people's opportunities actually determine what choices they have to make.[181]

In Philadelphia, people living in higher-income zip codes were tested at a rate six times greater than those in poor areas, according to an analysis done at Drexel University. A report from a Massachusetts-based biotech company, using patient surveys and hospital billing data from seven states in February and March 2020, showed African Americans who reported coronavirus symptoms were less likely to receive testing.[182]

The pandemic provided compelling evidence of the inequity and biases in our healthcare system. The actions that our country take in the next few months and years will determine if it has the resolve to make necessary changes. For the past few years, the government administration has departed from science and the tenets of truth, fairness, compassion and civility that provide the foundation for a democracy. Does our country want a better life for everyone? Or will we decide that certain groups of people don't matter? The results will define our country for at least a generation.

Abuse of Power by Bullying

According to a recent poll, 48 percent of children ages nine to thirteen years of age said they had been bullied; and 86 percent said they had seen someone else being bullied.[183] Today with children using technology such as cellphones and internet, the number has likely grown, and our concerns have expanded to "cyberbullying".

We focus special attention on this topic, not only because of its prevalence, but because it helps explain other forms of abuse of power, and why empowerment is important.

Bullying takes many forms:

- **Emotional bullying** is especially common among girls where victims may be shunned, excluded or made the subject of rumors.
- **Physical bullying** includes threats of physical harm which may accompany verbal threats and such physical acts as arm-twisting, striking and kicking.
- **Verbal bullying** includes name calling, mocking, and being the subject of jokes and/or negative nicknames.
- **Sexual bullying** is also known as sexual harassment and includes unwanted physical contact or sexually abusive and inappropriate comments.

- **Racist bullying** includes taunting and/or offensive gestures, and slurs aimed at an individual's racial background.

We have already suggested one reason for children becoming bullies: learning early the ability to control parents. Bullies typically target people that are different from themselves (overweight, a physical difference, or showing unique behaviors), and whom they believe are unlikely to retaliate.

Bullying may also be a learned behavior as a child's way of dealing with his/her own problems. If they came from families who practice name-calling, expressions of anger, and physical abuse, they copy what they have experienced.

Both the bully and the victim may have low self-esteem. The bully may appear to be stronger, more in control and thus more important and popular, but the bully is simply acting in accordance with unhealthy attitudes and beliefs held toward self and others.

The dangers of bullying have led to a striking rise in suicides among middle-school aged students. The suicide rate among the ten-to-fourteen-year-old demographic doubled between 2007 and 2014 surpassing the death rate from car crashes. The use of social media has increased the reach and unrelenting power of bullying. "With social media, you can't turn people off," said Phyllis Alongi, clinical director of the Society for the Prevention of Teen Suicide."[184]

Healthy Approaches to Dealing with Bullying

Is your child bullying other children? If you suspect your child is behaving like a bully, it is important to stay calm, not become angry or defensive, and talk in an authentic (disappointed, but not judgmental), empathic ("I need to understand"), manner that puts your child at ease. Ask your child questions that help you understand exactly what was done and what prompted the bullying behavior: "What happened?" "What feelings led to the outburst?" "Are there problems at home or at school?" "Was your action intentional?" "How do you feel about what has happened?"

Depending on the responses you receive, you may wish to speak to a school counselor or mental health professional, if you feel the need for more guidance. Possibly you may wish to reflect on the communication being practiced at home. For example, if your child is receiving name-calling and taunting from a sibling, he/she could be using these tactics against other children perceived as weak.[185]

In addition to modeling healthy (non-controlling) communication at home, here are some ways to encourage your child to cease bullying:

- Establish the rule that your family will not tolerate bullying behaviors. Rewards and punishments may need to be implemented. For example, if the child is cyber bullying, you take away access to the technologies that are being employed. Use the internet to research bullying and its effects, and then construct a plan of action.

- Insist that people who are different must be treated with respect.
- Observe your child interacting with other children. Are there patterns that reflect manipulation and control? Provide positive reinforcement when healthy communication is observed.
- Emphasize the unconditional love you have for your child. Try not to label your child a bully, instead talk about the act of bullying. Your disapproval is for the behavior, not for the child. Your child will recognize that behaviors can change.

As we discipline children, we must be careful to not bully or shame them. We teach them to be self-disciplined in safe, ethical ways that have predictable consequences. Finally, you may need to get outside help if behaviors don't change. The costs are too great to be ignored.

If you suspect your child is being bullied, they may be reluctant to admit it. Physical bullying may leave bruises, but less obvious new behaviors may be signs of a problem: missing money or belongings; poor concentration or irritability; less enthusiasm for school (increasing absences due to stomach aches); staying away from school activities; behavioral changes (bedwetting, headaches).

Being a victim of bullying can have long-term consequences including leading to substance abuse and withdrawal. Trust in future relationships may be more tentative, and the victim is more likely to experience depression and anxiety.[186]

There are ways you can help if you suspect he/she is being bullied. Be a good, empathic listener. It is important to show your love and support, since your child is feeling vulnerable. As you empathize, validate your child's feelings – don't minimize them. If you learn your child is being bullied, resist responding with anger or sadness; instead, reassure your child that he or she isn't to blame. Probe the circumstances, such as locations of the abuse and whether others are facing similar conditions.

Fighting back is rarely a good reaction, since it can serve to make matters worse. Instead, give your child these strategies to ward off bullies:

- **Control your emotional response**. Bullies want to have control over your emotions; if you show anger, the bully feels more powerful. Anger and violence will not help. Most importantly, do not resort to physical force.
- **Ignore the bully**. Look them in the eye and tell them to stop. Then walk away with your head held high and ignore any further taunts. Bullies thrive on the reactions they receive, so by walking away, or ignoring hateful email messages, you are showing that the bully has no control over you.
- **Talk about it with adults**. Teachers, principals, and counselors are available to provide support. Everyone needs to ask for help occasionally so be responsible for your own well-being.
- **Cultivate support**. Friends and buddies may also be being bullied. Be

willing to stand together and provide mutual support for one another in times of need. A positive group of peers can promote self-esteem and a more supportive environment.

These actions hopefully will make positive changes. As a parent, if your child's school doesn't have one, talk to the principal about starting an anti-violence program. The problem of bullying is too great to ignore.

Adult Bullying

Unfortunately, bullying behaviors do not vanish with coming of age. A 2016 study reported that workplace bullying is frighteningly common; almost 75 percent of employees surveyed had been affected by workplace bullying as either a target or a witness. It has been defined by the Workplace Bullying Institute: "Workplace bullying is repeated, health-harming mistreatment of one or more persons (the targets) by one or more perpetrators. It is *abusive* conduct that is: threatening, humiliating, or intimidating, or work-interfering, i.e., sabotage which prevents work from getting done.[187] One of the main differences between childhood bullying and workplace bullying is that it tends to be less physical and more verbal and psychological in nature. The harm is visibly subtle and may not be discerned by an observer. Power disparities characteristically exist when targets cannot successfully defend themselves.[188]

Another difference from childhood bullying is that the targets of workplace bullying, instead of being loners or perceived as being "different;" may be the most skilled workers and/or are threatening to the bully. The adult bully is skilled at manipulation and control and sees everything as a competition. Bullying is an attempt to gain and exert power, or at least to put forth a powerful image.

If such bullying is permitted to continue on the job, it can greatly damage the organization. Victims will experience loss of confidence, develop increased stress, and job performance will decline. Victims become more likely to leave the job due to the abuse. Such negative organizational gauges as turn-over rates, job absences, and lower profits can be tied directly to bullying. Similar outcomes are also the result of sexual harassment and racial discrimination.

Another type of bullying is less direct. Passive aggressive behaviors are frequently committed by individuals who want something but are unwilling to assume responsibility for their words, emotions, or actions. The twisted logic goes: If I foist decisions onto you, I can blame you for my unhappiness. Even worse, I can punish you for slights that only I perceive, by subjecting you to things that "are not my fault" because they "were out of my control." The passive aggressive individual frequently wants to **appear** nice at the cost of **being nice**. They hide hostility while relinquishing power, blaming others for their actions or circumstances and drive others crazy with all of the things that go wrong that are "beyond their control," so missing deadlines, "forgetting" to do things, or having outside obstacles keep them from meeting commitments are frequent behaviors. They seldom assume responsibility for their own behaviors or things that go wrong during group tasks. Passive aggressive people frequently talk behind other's backs rather than discuss issues of behavior, disagreements, or preferences.

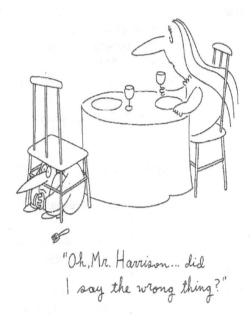

"Oh, Mr. Harrison... did I say the wrong thing?"

Communication Behaviors that Promote Empowerment

Your reactions to any given circumstance may or may not be empowering, (when you stand up for your rights without violating the rights of others), you respond with empowerment. Sometimes people who want to seem "nice" and "not cause trouble," permit greedy, dominant people to take advantage of them. They are not only cheating themselves, but also reinforcing the unfair, self-centered behavior of the manipulative person.

Empowerment, as was used in the Women's Movement in the 60's and 70's, is the act of declaring your personal preferences and defending your personal rights while respecting the differences and rights of others. The Women's Movement retained its societal influence by both having a major presence in the national news with marches, and rallies, and by building a behind-the-scenes network of influence in organizations and political support groups, as well as evaluating and developing women into leadership positions of power.

A young woman, Tarana Burke, proved to be the right person at the right time. In 2006, as a community organizer, she identified the phrase, "Me Too" as one that could help women. As someone who had experienced sexual assault herself, she wanted to help women and girls, especially those of color, who had also experienced and survived sexual violence.

She conceived the concept "empowerment through empathy." Within weeks the #MeToo movement exploded on Twitter, social media and major news outlets. The momentum accelerated, as more and more women told of their experiences and their truths, knowing that they weren't alone. As Tarana Burke tweeted: "It made my heart swell to see women using this idea – one we call 'empowerment through empathy,' to not only show the world how widespread and pervasive sexual violence is, but also to let other survivors know they are not alone."

Scholars also began to take note. Michelle Rodino-Colocino wrote an essay for a national communication journal in 2018, that considered whether Tarana Burke's #MeToo and *Time's Up* (a publication of the movement) "challenge the very systems of power that underlie harassment, discrimination, and assault by promoting empathy from the ground up (including individuals within our political-economic system)."[189]

One public effect of the movement was the accusations toward such well-known figures as Bill Cosby, Harvey Weinstein, Roger Ailes, Matt Lauer, and Kevin Spacey. Loss of jobs, public censure and legal proceedings followed. Others were accused and indicted and punitive action was not revealed.

In October 2018, Pew Research estimated that the #MeToo hashtag had been used approximately 19 million times on Twitter alone in the previous year, often by women and men who were inspired – in the wake of high-profile abuse allegations – to speak out about their own traumatic experiences.

Tarana Burke now heads #MeToo, an international movement in support of those who have experienced assault and harassment. Her experiences taught her lessons that resonate with many people working to prevent harm and improve health and health care around the world. We pass on four factors that Burke believes, promote empowerment.

1. **Rely on the power of empathy** – Empathy is a crucial component of effective person-centered care. Likewise, Burke believes "empowerment through empathy" is essential to her work. As she has said, "There's a difference between sympathy and empathy. Sympathy puts space between you and the other person, even though it's well-meaning. I can say: 'You experienced trauma, I'm so sorry that happened to you.' There's a space here between us. [By contrast], when we say, 'Me too,' that means there's something that draws you in. Even if for a moment, I get it. I see you, I hear you, I believe you. I connect with you."

2. **Improvement for the most vulnerable means to improve for all** – Health equity is essential. According to Burke, "The work of 'me too' builds on the existing efforts to dismantle systems of oppression that allow sexual violence, patriarchy, racism, and sexism to persist. We know that this approach will make our society better for everyone, not just survivors, because creating pathways to healing and restoration

moves us all closer to a world where everyone knows the peace of living without fear and the joy of living in your full dignity."

3. **Create joy to promote healing** – Restoring joy to the health care workforce is vital for improving health care. Joy is also part of the often-painful work Burke does, because it involves mutual support and collective action. "This is not really a movement about trauma," she has said. "It's a movement about joy. It's a movement about love and about respect, and it's about finding the ways that we can cultivate those things in our lives so that we can use them to combat the trauma we've experienced."

4. **Find strength in numbers** –It's validating and energizing to connect with others trying to challenge the status quo. As Burke has remarked, "Women have been speaking up for years about harassment and abuse. [This movement] has just created cover for those who didn't feel safe enough to speak up. The movement didn't create the concept of speaking out. It just allowed people to hear us better as a chorus and not a solo."[190]

In situations when you don't care to influence the outcome or have no investment, you may choose to be passive. When you respond aggressively or emotionally as in, "Hell, no!", you are at best insensitive and at worst bullies. Neither of these actions is empowered. Being empowered requires time and energy and vigilance.

Empowerment requires you to describe your feelings honestly, giving the reasons for your beliefs, and suggesting outcomes that you think are fair. Empowerment is thus based upon authenticity and empathy; it is truthful without exaggeration and is made with awareness of the feelings of the other.

We suggest that these are empowerment skills that illustrate healthy communication:

1. Describe your feelings using "I" statements which show you've taken responsibility for your feelings and personal needs: "I think_____;" "I feel _____ because_____."
2. Speak fluently and pleasantly. Uncertainty as shown by pauses may be interpreted as indecisiveness.
3. Describe the situation as you see it. Be as specific as possible. Stick to the "facts;" don't infer the motive of others.
4. Listen carefully to the other people and ask for clarification if you don't understand. Try to engage in open and honest dialogue.
5. Make clear requests of others. Don't expect them to guess what you want or intuit your needs. Honest discourse enhances the relationship.

Identify the empowerment skills that you use or would use if required. Such behaviors can be practiced with a trusted friend. A highly regarded book on this subject used by mental health professionals is: *Your Perfect Right.*[191]

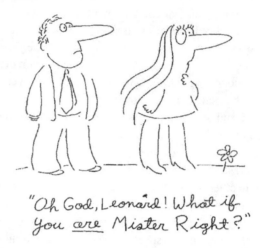

"Oh God, Leonard! What if you *are* Mister Right?"

In order to stand up for your rights, you must exercise empowerment, not to control others, but to control yourself and to influence that which is under your control for the strongest possible impact. As Americans, the basis for our political rights can be traced to our country's constitution. There is a difference between power over others and personal empowerment. Empowerment is the opposite of victimization. Empowerment means identifying and employing the power we hold in any circumstance including situations of oppression and powerlessness. The strong linkages between social class and health, show the dire consequences of powerlessness. In the next chapter, we address the importance of empowerment in healthy relationships.

Chapter 11 - Empowerment in a Healthy Relationship

Relationships are a crucial part of healthy living for everyone. Healthy relationships bring happiness rather than stress to those involved. We have already discussed some of the prerequisites for healthy relationships: people communicating authentically with one another and staying in touch with one another's feelings and perspectives. Trust, worth, receptiveness and mutual acceptance are constantly validated and reciprocated. For healthy relations to endure, each party will treasure the freedom of the other to be himself/herself and express his or her needs and desires openly without attempting to control the other (person).

The Development of Empowerment in a Relationship

Routinely you contact many new people at work, socially, and in all phases of your life. Most of these meetings are quickly over, and never to be furthered, but occasionally you meet a person with whom you wish to initiate a new relationship. According to a study in the 1970's, the first four minutes of a meeting with a person decide whether the connection will move in the direction of greater intimacy, or remain distant and impersonal.[192] During this time, the two people size up one another through mutual exploration, and determine what Giffin and Patton called "estimated relationship potential."[193] The two will mutually decide to continue to spend time together or to terminate the acquaintance. This agreement is based on both verbal and nonverbal communication (eye contact, future plans and exchanged information). Before deciding to prolong the acquaintance, each person must feel that the other person has attributes that can enrich his/her existence and fulfill personal needs. You have learned to be guarded in initial encounters. Your available time and energy are finite resources that force you to limit the number and amount of investment you allocate to new relationships.

The deepening of the relationship may cease at any point. For a healthy relationship to continue to develop between new friends, partners may negotiate either openly or covertly the terms of the friendship. The authentic and empowered individual asserts her or his needs. Partners who express their desires openly have a better chance of finding a partner willing to comply. Power and control issues must be resolved. Empowerment is a consciously developed behavior used in interpersonal relationships to mitigate control issues. Neither party attempts nor desires to control or force decisions on the other. There are many relationships in which one person hands over power to the other to make decisions for the couple. It is extremely difficult to maintain a healthy relationship under this circumstance. The partners may revert to impersonal stereotypical roles. Without copious ongoing communication, the powerful partner must guess desires and needs of the dependent party as he or she makes decisions, so needs of either or both parties may go unmet. Resentment can set in on the part of either or both partners. The goal of empowerment is truly shared decision-making. The ability to stay in growing relationships without diminishing, but rather expanding, one another's existence is what healthy relationships are about.

If a person is required to be dependent on someone who is controlling, overly critical, intimidating, and demeaning, the situation may give rise to stress, headaches, digestive upsets, and other symptoms of ill health. As Sidney Jourard has observed:

> Many physicians who have become alert to interpersonal sources of stress have been able to prove that for given patients, their symptoms of asthma, hemorrhoids, skin eruptions, hypertension, diarrhea, and so on, arose and lasted as long as the patient was inescapably involved with another person, and disappeared as soon as the relationship was ended.[194]

A relationship grows and deepens as a consequence of directly addressing conflicts and impasses head on and reconciling them. Interpersonal conflicts and impasses constitute problems that require solutions so that a healthy relationship may be maintained.

Conflict and Conflict Resolution

Whenever people encounter a problem in their everyday living, they vary their behavior until they find the changes that are successful in solving the problem. With no conflicts or impasses, there would be no incentives to change. If a person had no need to stay afloat and move in water, he/she would never learn to swim. If no one makes demands on you, you will never learn behaviors that please the other person. Conflict truly has a silver lining: it provides an opportunity for growth. In many ways, the opposite of love is not hate, but indifference. To engage in a conflict is a way of saying "yes" to the relationship's possibilities. Avoiding conflict indicates that the relationship is not worth the energy expended seeking resolution. It's an acceptance of "peace" at the cost of growth and joint-satisfaction.

As long as you act on the assumption that differences between persons are reason enough for conflict, you will be unhappy until partnered with a mirror. You might make unconscious demands that you want the person to be *like* you. Virginia Satir notes several such differences which may spark disagreement: wishes, habits, tastes, expectations, opinions, and religious beliefs.[195]

Even with high trust levels and self-esteem, joint living requires that some choices be made interdependently. What will you share or do separately? Unnecessary harm can come to the relationship, however, if either partner or both have such low self-esteem that every difference is seen as a repudiation of the other.

The choice to engage in conflict does not require the decision to fail, to destroy, or to win. In many ways, if either partner wins an argument while the other partner loses, the relationship suffers. A true win is a mutually agreed upon outcome that satisfies both parties.

Concern for the Growth and Welfare of the Other

In a healthy relationship, each participant is actively concerned for the welfare of the other. Each person wants the other to be well, happy, and growing. Because of deep-felt empathy, the satisfaction of the other person is felt as deeply as satisfaction for the self.

You may have noted that in the preceding narrative, we did not specify whether we were referring to friendships between partners/spouses of the same or of the opposite sex, or between members of the same family. Different expectations and behavioral norms guide each of these relationships, as well as differing degrees of commitment, but most of what has been said applies to all types of relationships. Your concern is to identify attitudes and behaviors that promote health and well-being for the people involved.

In a healthy relationship, each partner values the autonomy, development; and health of the other. Various degrees of conflict will certainly emerge. A wife who wishes to advance her education or return to the workplace may threaten a husband who is happy with the status quo. Parents may wish unwilling obedience and compliance from a child. In each case, if the wishes of one partner overrides those of the other, the quality of the relationship is at risk. Mutual respect is endangered.

Carl Rogers referred to the need for respecting another's individuality with "unconditional positive regard" as a necessary condition for mutual well-being. He stated, "Role and role expectations tend to drop away and are replaced by the person, choosing his/her own way of behaving.[196] Since Rogers' time, forced male and female stereotypic roles have been challenged, yet remain implicit in our society in issues such as wages, work expectations, insurance, birth control, parenting, and division of labor in the home. Authenticity and mutual empathy lay the groundwork for each party to empower the other.

In a healthy relationship, each partner respects the other's needs and desires. If one partner's choices violate the core values of the other, the relationship will be strained. A similar end is projected when one partner violates his or her own core values even if it's out of deference to the other. If a divorce, break-up of a friendship, moving from a parent's home, or resignation from a job is necessary for promoting growth and autonomy, the other person, in a healthy relationship will support this decision.

A key problem exists when both spouses have attractive opportunities for employment in different communities. Solving this problem demands frank discussions of personal goals, desires, dreams, and feelings. The couple must build a united vision and genuinely seek a way in which their separate wishes fit in that

124

greater one—a way for both partners to "win." Only after discovering that such a solution is not possible, should they consider compromise or sacrifice in order to meet their united vision.

As Rogers stated: "There is a more realistic appraisal of the needs each can meet in the other. When a man is thinking of his partner as a person, it becomes apparent that it is most unlikely that he can meet all of her needs. With equal force, it strikes the woman that she cannot be everything to the man."[197]

It becomes realistic to recognize that each partner in a healthy relationship needs to grant the other more time and living space for independent interests, outside relationships, and time alone. As Rogers, again states: "To the extent that each partner becomes truly a free agent, then the relationship only has permanence if the partners are committed to each other, are in good communication with each other, accept themselves as separate persons, and live together as persons, not roles."[198]

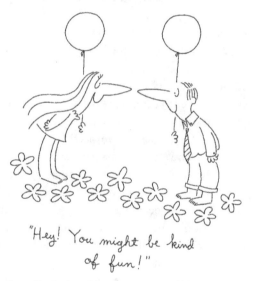

"Hey! You might be kind of fun!"

We remind you that all relationships are constantly in process, but the attributes that keep it moving in a healthy direction are mutual respect, trust, separateness, equality, honest communication, pleasure, and joy.

Nurturing Relationships During the Coronavirus Pandemic of 2020

The coronavirus outbreak dramatically changed our lives. Millions of us lost our normal ways of seeing others as we tried to keep each other safe. Many of us found ourselves spending far more time than we were used to with those who share our homes, whether family, housemates or both. For the first time since the early 19th century, many parents and children, and even grandchildren – were under the same roof all the time. These experiences of forced togetherness either deepened the relationship and built stronger connections – or produced a dynamic that felt dangerous or intolerable. Before considering the unhealthy relationships, let's look at the healthy ones.

We know, for example, that the U.S. divorce rate plummeted during the Great Depression and the 2008 financial crash. Brad Wilcox, Director of the National Marriage Project at the University of Virginia, observed: "When society is facing a tremendous challenge or there's a big uptick in suffering, people orient themselves in a less self-centered way and in a more family-centric way.[199]

Several families reported that they grew closer, bonding more deeply as they rode out the pandemic and began to function as a team. Families that grew closer and supported one another shared some factors that helped them utilize their time in productive ways:

- They scheduled and agreed on a time each day when everyone could say how they were feeling. They tried to share and listen without judgment, and were reminded that in this stressful and anxious time people may be more irritable than usual.
- They agreed on who is using which parts of the home and when. People were allowed personal space for reading, resting, or just being alone.
- Household tasks such as cooking and cleaning were shared and traded. Having a daily routine helped everyone to feel more in control.
- Some families devised creative, educational uses of time, such as more hands-on activities in art and music than before; one family built an entire LEGO-based trade economy, while another said they spent less time on mechanics and "more time together."[200]

Providing schooling, recreation and bonding between multiple generations deepened relationships in these for years to come.

Unhealthy Relationships

In 2014, The Hall Mental Health Center at Washington University, St. Louis, distributed a useful checklist and analysis that enumerated signs and behaviors in unhealthy relationships. As we have suggested, such relationships cause stress, and lead to numerous health problems:

- **Attempting to change a partner by manipulation**. When manipulation becomes the usual mode of interacting with the significant other, it is a serious sign of impaired mental health. It implies, among other things, a distrust of the other person leading to alienation and contempt. The manipulated partner learns to suppress spontaneous feelings leading to self-alienation.[201] The manipulated partner, often without conscious awareness, becomes whatever the other person likes, and then pretends to be the kind of person who behaves that way. Sydney Jourard has observed:

  The major factor responsible for habitually contrived interpersonal behavior is the belief, conscious or implicit, that to be one's real self is dangerous; that exposure of real feelings and motives will result in rejection or ridicule. Such a belief stems from experiences of punishment and rejection at the hands of parents and other significant persons. To avoid punishment in the future, the child represses his real self in interpersonal situations and learns to become a contriver, an "other-directed" character. Of course, more serious outcomes are possible too: neurosis, psychopathic personality, and psychosis.[202]

- **The partners begin to feel the need to justify their actions** – what they do and whom they see. Pressure is felt to cease activities that had once been enjoyable. One or both partners worries if they disagree with the other.
- **The partners create separate social networks**. They choose to spend less and less time with one another. They have fewer common friends and have a lack of respect for each other's friends and family.
- **Their sex lives suffer**. One partner feels pressured and even forced to have sex. They may cease to be concerned about the other's pleasure and satisfaction, and may deny the use of birth control.
- **They experience physical abuse**. One partner may resort to yelling or physical violence during an argument. Such abuse includes: intimidation (making a partner afraid by using looks, actions, or gestures that imply danger); threats and manipulation (making statements that instill fear; threatening harm to the partner or the children, or to self); and economic abuse (concealing financial information; making the partner have to ask or beg for money).

Obviously, these signs vary in the degree to which they threaten the continuation of the relationship, but usually demand professional help and assistance. Repeated violations of one partner by the other are a clear sign that it is an unhealthy relationship that possibly needs to be ended.

The Gottman Institute was started in 1976 to study married couples to better understand why some marriages end quickly and others endure for long periods. Dr. John Gottman teamed with Dr. Robert Levenson to first study married couples engaged in conflict, utilizing psycho-physiological measurements of heart rate, blood pressure, and gross motor activity. In a major longitudinal study, the researchers studied 3,000 couples for 20 years.[203] They compared couples who maintained or grew in the "level of happiness" in their marriage, and those who deteriorated in the happiness level to the extent that the marriage ended. The number of years they stayed together was closely associated with happiness and positive feelings expressed in the relationship. The researchers found that the more physiologically aroused in all channels the couples were, the more their marriages deteriorated. For these couples, conflict produced physical reactions similar to the fight/flee emotional responses to danger.

Early divorces were attributed to what Gottman termed the "Four Horsemen" – criticism, contempt, defensiveness and stonewalling. Couples who stayed together during and after the conflicts shared behaviors that avoided putdowns of each other, showed nonverbal demonstrations of affirmation, and validation of one another. These couples also shared humor, made remarks of affection and showed empathy for their partner, even in conflict. Homosexual couples were not significantly different from heterosexual couples in the Gottman research data.[204]

EFFECT OF THE 2020 PANDEMIC IN UNHEALTHY RELATIONSHIPS

For some people, such as those living with domestic violence or abuse, staying home during the pandemic was dangerous or intolerable. Consider the problem for some families; with over 30 million unemployed; people still going to work in critical industries and essential jobs faced the possibility of being infected daily and were putting in longer hours than usual – not only spending less time at home but also having to deal with childcare crises or the care of elderly or ill family members. Millions of families had to deal with losses of loved ones, jobs and income, which produced such stress as to harm people's marriages and disrupt family life.

The director of the National Violence Hotline said that their staff, working remotely, urged people in "potentially risky situations" to formulate a personal safety plan. Using a more discreet chat and text option available on their website, the counselors advised setting up a scheduled call with relatives or trusted friends and possibly setting up a code phrase to signal an emergency that required help.[205] Victims spent night and day trapped at home with their abusers with tensions rising, nowhere to escape and no idea if it would end.

With child abuse cases already totaling approximately three million each year, and many more going unreported, many deep emotional and mental wounds are created. Incidences of violence against women and children especially has increased. Examples of emotional abuse and neglect include name-calling, verbal insults, yelling, abandonment, or failure to provide adequate shelter, medical care, and nutrition. At the time of the pandemic, the increased stress levels among parents proved to be significant predictors of physical abuse, verbal abuse and neglect.[206]

Empowering Your Partner with Pleasure and Happiness

Good relational health promotes longer, more fulfilling lives. One of the greatest joys can come in the form of enjoying pleasures and bringing joy to one another. As we pointed out in our discussion of the evolution of the human brain, health-promoting behaviors are biologically connected to positive feelings. Pleasures, from caring for others to listening empathetically to someone in need, guides us to better health.[207]

Our American work ethic can get in the way of allowing ourselves to play and to seek personal and relational pleasures. We may be taught to feel guilty if we consciously seek pleasure. Such activity is viewed as "unproductive." In truth, fun and play can promote genuine health that results in greater productivity. Don't be a slave to the work ethic! Unfortunately, many religions view pleasure, especially that which involves sensuality, as morally corrupting. As physicians suggest, "our health, happiness, and future depend upon understanding and reversing this deeply rooted cultural denial of pleasure and leisure. Sensitivity and spirituality need not conflict."[208]

One of the greatest areas of pleasure is in a healthy relationship where each partner has the capacity to feel and demonstrate love for each other. In such relationships, partners are not ashamed or afraid to let their needs and desires be known to the other. Each wants to please the other and promote their happiness.

Be good to yourself and to your significant others: whether it's an enjoyable meal out, a glass of beer or wine, a well-deserved foot-rub, a day in the park, or a long pleasurable cruise. Research has shown that laughter can raise pain thresholds and make your immune system more active in a positive way. Laughter has been shown to boost the levels of antibodies in saliva that help defend against infections like colds.[209]

Encourage your partner to seek pleasure and satisfaction without having to feel guilty. In the healthy relationship, each partner identifies closely with the needs and feelings of the other. When this occurs, the satisfactions of the other are felt as deeply as satisfaction for the self.

LAUGHTER, PLEASURE AND HEALTH

Happiness, pleasure and laughter between partners is reciprocal. Sharing with a significant other heightens the feelings and the joy. Allowing yourselves to feast upon fun and pleasure will foster positive emotional connections. A 2015 study found that laughter subconsciously increased people's willingness to self-disclose, leading to greater feelings of affection.[210]

Laughter has been regularly promoted as a source of health and well-being. Professor Robin Dunbar, an evolutionary psychologist at Oxford, studied this phenomenon in 2011. He found that the physical act of laughing, that is, the simple muscular exertions, trigger an increase in endorphins. Shared laughing contributes to closeness and bonding, according to Dunbar.[211]

Your moods have both negative and positive influence on your health. Grief has been shown to induce stress hormones that suppress the immune functions leading to a greater risk of sickness. Laughter appears to shut down the release of stress hormones like cortisol, and trigger the release of dopamine which has calming, anti-anxiety benefits. The health benefits of laughter range from lowered levels of inflammation to improved blood flow. One research study compared the positive benefits of laughter to such positive lifestyle activities as good diet, exercise and good sleep.[212]

Dr. Robert Provine, a neuroscientist at the University of Maryland, has stated that you are thirty times more likely to laugh around other people than you are by yourself, another benefit of social relationships. As Provine states, "When we laugh, we're in a happy place. That's always a good thing."[213]

Your attitudes toward guilt-free pleasure and the freedom to let go and enjoy yourself are crucial. A balance must be maintained between self-regulation to prevent overindulgence, and need-fulfilling rewards to bring pleasures. When you wake up in the morning, focus on your breathing and your body and think of having another day to enjoy. Smile because researchers have discovered even forced smiles activate the chemicals in your brain that elevate your mood.[214] Connect with the positive and rewarding aspects of your life that make you happy and comfortable: your cup of coffee, the presence of a loved one, the morning newspaper and the birds singing. Think of happy memories. You may wish to make a list of activities or events that make you happy. Perhaps it's accomplishing tasks around the house, exercising, writing, creative activities, sports, helping others, talking to friends, or going to the theatre. Plan your day by rewarding yourself with those activities that you look forward to doing.

Psychologist Robert Ornstein and physician David Sobel argue that, "Pleasure rewards us twice: first in immediate enjoyment and second in improved health".[215] They reported that the healthy, robust people who lead high quality lives in their study, more consistently reported a positive attitude than adherence to current health professional's recommendations. Much of their success comes from their attitude. They wrote:

> The positive moods and pleasurable expectation of healthy people were so striking to us that we began to collect experiences of what these people were like. As a rule, they were optimistic and happy no matter their difficulties. They enjoyed small simple pleasures and stolen moments: witnessing the sunrise, building a model classic car, or indulging in silly talk with their spouses, kids, and pets. Surprisingly to us, they highlighted minor things that pleased them; a shotgun collection, playing the violin passionately (though terribly), or cooking their favorite meals. These pursuits seemed somehow to absorb some of the troubles of their active lives.[216]

They summarize by saying, "In short, the healthiest people seem to be pleasure-loving, pleasure seeking, pleasure-creating individuals."[217] You won't go far wrong if you pursue healthy pleasures. What could be more welcomed advice?

SOCIAL RELATIONSHIPS AND HEALTH

As we have previously suggested, there is a growing recognition of the connection of social relationships to health and well-being throughout life. In 2001, Dr. Teresa Seeman, Professor of Medicine and Epidemiology at UCLA, summarized a large body of research that showed consistent association between quality of social life and longevity and mental health. She reported associations between higher reported levels of support and better physiological profiles (lower heart rate, lower systolic blood pressure, lower serum cholesterol, and lower urinary epinephrine).[218]

According to Seeman, the primary pathway that links the social world to internal physiology is the cognitive and emotional processing in the brain that influences neuroendocrine arousal. Positive or negative relational reactions lead directly to positive or negative physiological functioning. She labels this the "double-edged sword" of social relationships that either help or hinder all aspects of health. Her work provides valuable insight into how social relationships "get under the skin" to directly affect health and resistance to disease.

The quality of your relationships affects you on a health continuum in the same way as other choices you make: good nutrition versus bad nutrition; exercise versus no exercise; healthy foods versus fast food. One choice leads to longer, happier and more fulfilling lives, while the alternative leads in the opposite direction.

Poverty and lower socioeconomic status limit a person's health choices. Obviously, public health policies that broaden choices promote empowerment for citizens. Parents should not have to choose between providing their children with food or with health care. In the next chapter, we will address this issue of empowerment in our society.

Neuroscientists have repeatedly found that relationships affect the brains of people who are in supportive, mutually satisfying relationships. Studies of longevity, medical and mental health, happiness, and intelligence give compelling evidence of healthy, supportive relationships.

Personal Reflections

Reflect on several of your relationships: parent-child, boss-employee, close friend. How healthy are they? What role does power play?

What has been your family history in terms of gender roles? Compare your parents' division of labor with your own relationships. Do you feel comfortable within your relationships with work assignments? If not, plan to adjust, and share your planned changes with those affected.

Chapter 12 - Healthy Decision Making in Our Society

History is a record of many oppressive social and political systems in which people have been exploited in cruel, dehumanizing ways. Healthy lives require enlightened perspectives in society's decision making that allow people to reach their full potential. Life, liberty, and the pursuit of happiness are perquisite goals for any civilized society. Throughout history, people have had to act courageously and intelligently to improve their situations.

Fortunately, we live in a democratic society in which checks and balances are provided to maintain orderly processes of decision making through voting. No society, however, is ever perfect in its processes or procedures for achieving the greatest good for the maximum of its citizens. In this chapter, we will build upon the information from the previous chapters and present our plans for promoting healthier societal decision making.

The Process of Societal Changes

In the nineteenth century, a fundamental transition occurred in our society when the agrarian economy was superseded by the industrial economy. Many theories and practices, procedures and organizational structures of modern management, and governments were formulated during that period of transition and the Industrial Age that evolved. The practices were modernized by twentieth century improvements and by new technology designed to improve their efficiency. But at heart there remained the vestiges of earlier times. As we are engaged in a shift to the Information Age, a key lesson can be learned from the last transition. The underlying technology both enables and pushes the transition. For the Industrial Age, the steam engine, internal combustion engine, and jet engine sequentially drove technology development. In the Information Age, the emergence of computing, the fusing of telecommunications with computers, and the emergence of ubiquitous networking have driven the transition to the new information-based economy. The term "social media" is now widely used to designate a blend of communication that is both personal and mediated.

New generations of powerful applications create both opportunities and challenges. There are at least three fundamental ways in which today is converting tomorrow into a world that will not resemble yesterday. These three themes – rate and magnitude of change, interrelatedness of people, and continuing escalation of human aspirations – can be viewed as challenges we must meet.

Rate and Magnitude of Change

Social and technological changes have accelerated to the point that the old adage of "waiting to see what happens" no longer applies. We must develop new strategies for living with change, for anticipating problems, and for designing creative alternative solutions. The faster you go, the greater the lead time you need to recognize trends, prepare solutions, and revise your course of action.

Consider the following travel analogy. If you drive an automobile down the road at twenty-five miles an hour, you can leisurely watch for signs and landmarks; you can turn off at the last minute. If, however, you are driving at seventy-five miles an hour, you have to be more alert to exits ahead. In other words, you need early warning systems as you anticipate the amount of change in your future. Our world includes too many people, too many decisions, and too much information. We have constant sensory overload. One expert has suggested that recorded knowledge doubled between the years 1 AD and 1750; another doubling occurred between 1750 and 1900; a third between 1900 and 1950; a fourth between 1950 and 1960; and a fifth between 1960 and 1963. Since then, knowledge is said to be doubling approximately every six months. In this world of quantitative overload, it is easy to lose perspective and become disoriented.

Electronic media has added to the information overload. Periods of time away from a desk result in a deluge of e-mail messages. Unfortunately, not all the information distributed is accurate or useful. You cannot trust all information, and the need to differentiate between the accurate and the inaccurate is crucial. For example, erroneous information regarding negative side effects of childhood vaccinations has resulted in needless deaths. Repetitive statements are persuasive and if we are not careful, we accept them over scientifically verified facts. False statements remain false regardless of the number of times they are repeated and regardless of the volume at which they are announced. It is sad that repetition and vehemence increase a person's willingness to believe. This tendency is one of the reasons that viral lies are so insidious.

The ways that a person can perceive change are many and subjective. For the harried and harassed, additional change may represent threatening pressure. For the bored, change may create appealing excitement. In terms of the magnitude of change, "more" has no absolute value and is not necessarily good nor bad. The real question is "more of what?" To most of us, more income is good, but more bills are bad, and the difference between the two may determine happiness or unhappiness. There's nothing inherently threatening or frightening in the increase of the number of things or options in our environment.

Expanded awareness has always been a major thrust in the evolution of humankind. In studies on child development, for example, we call home environments *rich* when they have ample sources of stimulation, *poor* when there are few. Psychological experiments on sensory deprivation have demonstrated that the human nervous system may become seriously disoriented when removed from normal sense excitements, a situation analogous to the withholding of nourishment from the physical body. Human experiences will continue to be enriched by greater interaction with people and places. Radio, television, computers, and satellites have put us in touch with the remote, the strange, and the previously inaccessible. Through electronic communication, our senses are connected directly with the rest of our globe and with outer space. The connections help us take the halting but vital steps toward feeling a unity with the rest of our globe.

The opportunities provided by technological advances in social media, science, and health bring threats as well. We increasingly have the power to make decisions that we have no reverse. Paths we take may never be retraced. Biologically, we can remake the human species, but behind our capacities for genetic engineering lurk the threats of the monster suggested in the story of Dr. Frankenstein. Who is wise enough to decide what should be done and how will it be decided? The same questions are present in nuclear physics and technology, through which it is possible to devastate our entire planet. And, in a more immediate sense, how do we confront the issue of terrorism? We know that fanatics have the power to blow up cities and contaminate public water supplies. These are not pleasant thoughts, but we must improve our odds at anticipating the problems and planning our responses. The worst crises are those for which we are unprepared and which surprise us. September 11, 2001 marked a wake-up call for our country. The toll exacted by the COVID 19 pandemic on our physical and psychological welfare, the loss of life, suffering and long-term effects are yet to be determined.

Interrelatedness of People

No longer is it possible to be separate or isolated from other people. The world and its people form one gigantic system. What goes on in any one place in some way affects every other place. The ecological model is universal. We are all members of and served by complex systems. Some of these are systems of nature, some are massive human organizations, and some are huge technological systems. Self-sufficiency in our society has diminished and dependency has increased. One of the consequences in government has been a tendency toward more and more regulation to the point that many suggest is over-regulation. Threats of pollution and nuclear explosions are global in potential impact. There is no place to hide. The pandemic verified this reality.

Most of the problems we face today are people-made problems. The solutions we find will be people-made solutions. Our achievements in science and technology have contributed both to the problems and to the potential solutions. Pollution is a worldwide threat that cannot be denied; population pressures and food shortages have global implications. As we have suggested, communication and transportation technologies have brought all parts of the world into direct contact with each other. However, much of our thinking from past models is parochial and provincial; most of our habits and our institutions are based on models from earlier ages.

We instinctively compete with each other and define "winning" as ending up with more than our neighbors. It is important to note that the world has changed.

In the future, winning will be measured by how successfully you can make the world work for everybody. The real enemies will *not* be other people but will be starvation, disease, illiteracy, climate change, and terrorism. The world will be run as a whole, or not run at all. Cooperation is a necessity, not a luxury. We are in a race between our old instincts and the new demands of our global culture.

Our process perspective tells us that any human act sends ripples across the entire human pond. All of us are affected by the problems that affect any nation. No national wall is high enough to shield you from the difficulties that affect your neighbors. We may talk of self-sufficiency in energy resources, for example, but no nation can be truly self-sufficient in a world that is crowded, finite, and closely connected. To use an old cliché, we are all passengers on Spaceship Earth. Either we learn to live and share with each other, or we will wreck the vehicle before we travel much farther into the orbit of the future. To use another metaphor, we are one large family on a summer's vacation in a camper. Either we learn to get along in limited space and with limited supplies, or we ruin the trip. The only alternative to compromise is chaos. Our figurative family can always call it off and turn back, but our world doesn't have that choice. We can either go forward on a short and disastrous trip, or a long journey in harmony through time and space.

The pandemic of 2020 illustrated the metaphor as groupings of people were forced to choose between cooperation and chaos. A clear correlation was shown in a country's choice and the number of the cases, the spread of the virus, and the deaths occurring.

Continuing Escalation of Human Aspirations

Human beings all over the world long for more satisfying lives. Some of the longings are material, such as for food, medical care, and a higher standard of living. Many of the longings are spiritual and ethical: rights of personal dignity, political autonomy, and religious freedom, including the "freedom from religion." The crucial change, however, has been the shift from a mere longing to an expectation. In the latter part of the twentieth century, hopes and wishes were replaced by demands and insistences. The reason was an expanded sense that humankind can do better if it so wishes, and people of the world are not simply helpless victims tossed on waves of chance. A second contributing factor has been the effect of the mass media. Through television's window of the world, underdeveloped countries and deprived masses could see and envy varying degrees of affluence in the lifestyles of the "rich and famous."

As with the other dimensions, the expectations explosion has both positive and negative features. Both human philosophy and human experiences are centered on a few major counterpoints. For example, good and bad; right and wrong; war and peace; truth and untruth; beauty and ugliness. As governments and societies have evolved, one key counterpoint has always been the individual and the group, or sometimes the individual versus the group. This is a recurring issue in national political matters with the rising expectations of the world population.

What rights should an individual have that transcend the rights of the group? What rights should the group have to control the behavior of the individual? Diverse cultures and political regimes have given different answers to these questions over time, and these different answers have ignited wars and revolutions. For nations and for individuals, development has three phases. For clarity, we will use the frame of game-playing to illustrate our points. The first phase of any game is *how to play*. A young child raises this question as they watch brothers and sisters bat balls or shoot baskets. "Can I play? Show me how." Our young nation had the same problem 250 years ago, and we learned fast. The second phase of any game is *how to win*. After a while, just playing is not enough. The youngster learns to score points, do well, and beat other players. This is the spirit of competition. It is a strong motivator and helps to sharpen skills. Once again, the same is true for nations. In our nation, capitalism is synonymous with innovation, enterprise, economic competition in the private sector, etc. Our captains of industry have won in the marketplace because they have the same motivations as our best athletes.

It is also true that some of our captains of industry, political leaders and athletes have been known to cut corners here and there, and to put winning ahead of ethics. Thus, we come to the third phase of any game – *how to keep the game fair*. The real question today and in the future, is how to preserve the game and keep it fair for all players. Some social games have been rigged or fixed in the past, with unfair rules for women, black people, and other minorities. Many of us are unwilling to accept these rules any longer, and we will no longer accept the uncontrolled freewheeling and free dealing by unethical leaders in any of our professions.

In order for our society to be all that we aspire to, we must mindfully monitor our actions and interactions, being ever aware of the choices we have in any circumstances and the potential consequences.

Societal Goals Needed for a Healthier World

Consider for a moment the United States motto: **E pluribus Unum:** "Out of many, one." In the Declaration of Independence, our country established a challenging ethical goal: liberty and justice for all. This challenge is perhaps more difficult today in the light of political polarization and disagreement on basic values.

The father of one of your authors grew up on a Texas farm and had limited education. Yet he had a wise insight learned from life that he often repeated: "Everybody does better when everyone does better." We believe that this guideline is still a truism that provides a sound basis for societal decision making.

To move beyond where we are and begin to constructively address the problems that are undermining our societal health, we need to agree on certain goals based upon common values and common aspirations.

At the heart of the discontent and anger in our current society is the feeling that it is no longer "our" system. Many Americans seem to feel that there has been a "hostile takeover" of our electoral and governmental processes by powerful politicians, big-money contributors, and lobbyists who have little concern for middle class working people. Town hall meetings in congressional districts have been well attended by angry and exasperated voters who feel left out of the important decision-making process.

Yet at the heart of the public's negative feelings is something positive: Americans want to be involved in the politics and governing of our country. More and more people are pressing for empowerment. It appears that America's grassroots are alive with progressive agitation and greater political participation. Some people who had written off national politics as a "public relations charade" are now devoting time and energy to public service, and are looking for ways to influence national decisions such as those regarding health care.

We suggest and propose five principles that would guide us to a healthier society and world. We recognize that differences will exist between reasonable people about how to operationalize these guiding principles. Nevertheless, we believe that all citizens must share common goals and targets.

1. **Acceptance and respect for the interdependent process of all existence.**

    As we have emphasized, we are "all in this together." We need to resist the tempting policies that weaken others for selfish personal gain. We must pursue policies that permit everyone to be valued and empowered. We can no longer attempt to "win" at the expense of others. "Winning" needs to be thought of as a team effort involving the entire world. Rejoining the Paris Climate agreement was one step in the right direction to not squandering the many resources for which we are stewards.

2. **Recognition and acceptance for the inherent worth and dignity of every single person on earth.**

    The rights of life including health, liberty and the pursuit of happiness must be available and extended to all people, everywhere. We must be champions of human rights throughout the world. We have a long way to go to make this goal a reality, but we need to have the goal in order to take the steps to make it happen.

3. **Support for a free and responsible search for reality, truth, meaning, and the rights of conscience for all persons.**

    Scientific research must be respected and applied for the health and well-being of humankind. We must resist censorship and limits on our capacity to access and share information and engage in democratic processes. Freedom of inquiry, expression of all ideas, and the press must be preserved and strengthened throughout the world. Resistance to science must be eradicated by education and advocacy.

4. **Trust, equity, fairness, and compassion in all human relationships.**

   Such values enrich every relationship and should be encouraged by support and empowerment. Laws, rules, and policies must encourage such behaviors. Our world leaders must endorse and model these principles. Humanity must learn to be humane.

5. **The goal of a world community with peace, liberty and justice for all.**

   The achievement of this goal is perhaps the most controversial and the most difficult to accomplish. We believe, however, that while this goal is Utopian, it is none-the-less, the only viable, long-term method for a world to succeed and continue to foster a healthy environment for its inhabitants.

We suggest that these five principles provide a fundamental basis for an American identity as we assert our interests in the global community. We encourage our citizens to take an active role by being empowered to influence the on-going debate. The decisions made will shape the moral fabric of the nation and will have a tremendous impact on our national identity as we interface with other nations in an increasingly globalized world.

The U.S. can be a model for the rest of the world by demonstrating the principles and showing the possibilities and the results. Perhaps we should use one of the principles for a year to guide citizens in understanding them and be able to visualize how the world could be with specific changes.

Given the impact of the COVID-19 pandemic on human health and the economy, there is concern that politicians will use the country's fears to enact draconian change to "keep America safe." That path could include policies to punish the countries we blame for the outbreak, abolishing the World Health Organization, protectionist trade policies in reaction to American trade deficits, actions to restore our country's "competitiveness," and less resistance to a military-run government. The country is split so deeply along partisan and value lines, that effective governing by either party is difficult to accomplish. Violence may escalate as the use of guns to challenge authority in the name of "patriotism "persists.

There is an alternate path based on our cited principles. Americans have been calling for the U.S. to once again be a global leader on issues of human health and well-being, and President Biden has responded. This action is based on making changes at home. It means restructuring our economic system from one that rewards only growth, to one that provides workers the support needed to be both productive and healthy. Reforms in industry and transportation are proposed to ensure that we don't need to be under lockdown to have clean air. The fight against climate change has been renewed and must be intensified with urgency.

The country that we envision after the coronavirus wake-up call, will again invest in the public services, programs and research that can protect human health and well-being for all citizens, not only in times of emergency, but all the time. We would restructure our economy to provide the public resources necessary for national preparedness and resilience. President Biden needs support to enact and fund his extensive agenda.

Beware being scared off by the words "socialized medicine." Try to recognize the scope of problems in healthcare that our country is attempting to deal with. Perhaps much of the world is right when they say that universal health care should be a universal right for all people.

We believe that ensuring that all people in the U.S. have affordable healthcare coverage and providing a defined set of health benefits, will move our country toward a healthier, more productive society. Additionally, our healthcare system must be able to account for and address social determinants such as socioeconomic status, housing, and occupational conditions, food availability, and environment that have a profound impact on health outcomes and costs.

The healthcare for all plans that we envision would emphasize the centrality of *primary care* and help to redesign the system of delivery and simplify the billing, expand the use of lower tier of medical expertise to initially screen patients to determine the best means to achieve their goals. The successful practices in other countries that have achieved excellent results with fewer resources should be reviewed and added to the plan.

The briefest looks at America's health crisis show how beneficial this change would be. The US continues to spend the most on healthcare per person per year of any country on earth. According to CDC data (2018), the ten countries that spent the most on healthcare per person were the following: US, $10,586, Switzerland, $7,317, Norway, $6,187, Germany, $5,980, Sweden, $5,447, Austria, $5, 395, Denmark, $5,299, Netherlands, $5,288, Luxembourg, $5,070, Australia, $5,005.[219] But the US is unique in that most healthcare is paid through private insurance and out-of-pocket costs.

America has been attempting to improve healthcare for decades yet has encountered blockages and lack of agreement on what constitutes improvement. This book has been our attempt to get there. We believe that personal usage and societal development of the three keys will help change our personal attitudes, goals and actions and focus on the societal conversation that needs to take place before nationwide action can occur. Americans are primed for such discussions. MEDIFIND, a consumer centered organization focused on information and ideas to improve healthcare, noted in 2021, that only 7 percent of all Americans are satisfied with the current healthcare system.[220] As Attorney Mary Gerisch has noted on behalf of the American Bar Association,

> In the United States, we cannot enjoy the right to health care. Our country has a system designed to deny, not support, the right to health. The United States does not really have a health care system, only a health insurance system. Our government champions human rights around the world, insisting that other

countries protect human rights, even imposing sanctions for
failure to do on. Our government is not as robust in protecting
rights at home.[221]

On July 20, 2021, the United States Center for Disease Control and Prevention released its yearly findings on health from 2020 and estimates for 2021. Life expectancy in the U.S. dropped the most years in the "Year of Death" category since WWII. The first year of the pandemic marked the sixth year in a row that life expectancy had declined. For 2020, the decline was in all ethnic and gender categories. [222]

Dr. Noreen Goldman, Director of Demography and Public Affairs at Princeton University stated: "It's staggering and depressing. The U.S. lags behind virtually all high-income countries and now its lagging further behind.[223] Despite this country's vast economic expenditures, its strong science research programs (evidenced by the development of three successful vaccines for COVID-19), U.S. health has been declining in relation to other advanced nations and our own past." Goldman goes on to touch on many of the health issues that first instigated this book's development.

....physical activity has declined with teenagers now spending
time on cellphones, videos and other electronic devices rather
than exercising. Many adults, as well as teenagers appear to
be stressed out as reflected by reliance on addictive drugs,
numbers of suicides, sleep-deprivation, heart attacks and
strokes, depression, anger issues, and other behavioral problems.
Unhealthy relationships have been shown to be toxic to the
participants. Above all, America is wavering in its core values,
resulting in polarization, absence of trust, reduction in health
safeguards, and increased international tension.[224]

One of the advantages of a universal healthcare system in the U.S. is the opportunity to address the epidemic level of non-communicable chronic diseases such as cardiovascular disease, type II diabetes, and obesity that strain our current economy by providing care for the currently uninsured and largely unhealthy segment of the U.S. population. Prevention programs can save money. For example, investing in community-based programs aimed at combatting physical inactivity, poor nutrition, and smoking could save the economy billions of dollars. Another recent analysis suggests that if 18 percent more U.S. elementary school children participated in 25 minutes of physical activities three times per week, the savings from medical costs and productivity would collectively be enormous.

Despite sizable economic costs upfront, we will reduce the unhealthy costs of an unhealthy country. The health disparities that were so transparent during the pandemic will be eliminated as universal healthcare will facilitate the necessary changes. The plan will encourage sustainable, preventive health practices and be advantageous for long-term public health as well as our economy. Most importantly, by recognizing the human right to healthcare, our country will be closer to one envisioned by our forefathers and responsive to the U.N. list of universal rights.

We need unifying leadership with an understanding of the unprecedented challenges facing us, including income inequity, class favoritism, the needs of emerging nations, and demanding dictators. In a national column on May 9, 2020, in advance of the presidential election, Kathleen Parker articulated the hope of most of us.

> "America has generally been lucky throughout its history: When faced with an existential crisis, the nation has somehow miraculously produced the kind of president – Washington, Lincoln, Franklin Roosevelt – who has, in the face of a do-or-die challenge, built a bridge to the future. Americans hunger for an aspirational message of unity and optimism. Or, as another president put it, hope and change."[225]

The authors believe that we have an optimistic future if we make the difficult but necessary decisions.

Promoting Human Evolution Through Self-Regulation

We have described empowerment, the means of attaining power, as the process by which relatively powerless people work together to increase control over events that determine their lives and health. For better decision making, we need improved behavioral training and continued brain exercises to promote the evolution of the human brain.

So where do you go from here? What are your alternatives? We believe that there are only three possible directions. First, we can wait and watch and to see what happens. Second, we can escalate our efforts at control and regulation. Third, we can start trying to reinvent human nature.

The first alternative is no answer at all; it is a tragic spectator sport; we have been a crisis society for too long – waiting until the disaster comes, then trying to figure out a remedy. We must switch to an anticipatory strategy. The risk is too great to rely on the old wait-and-see approach; we must aim at prevention. The controls and regulations from the second alternative may indeed be indispensable as stop-gap measures in a scary world – but new and greater ingenious threats will emerge and could spiral into a type of police state. Thus, we believe that the third alternative is the only viable one – the one that seems the most unrealistic on first examination. Is it possible to change "human nature"?

Fortunately, the exploding neuroscience research of the last two decades gives us perspective and directions for evolving human nature. Throughout the book we have been tracing the evolution of the human brain. We have repeatedly emphasized the differences between the two processing systems: the automatic response, our oldest system that responds to danger, and the reflective response that is the most recent to develop and the most sophisticated.

Neuroscience has introduced us to a third response system that has been labeled *controlled response*. This middle-ground system is based on self-regulation and controls that can be used to override automatic responses before they prove harmful.

Take, for example, your habits. You have developed automatic responses to recurring life situations that permit you to cope, feel better momentarily, and reduce stress; such coping habits become addictive, and you lose consciousness of other choices. Sam grew up in a chaotic household and found eating provided an escape and reduced his feelings of stress. "Comfort food" became an easy and available escape from daily stress at school and subsequently at work. Eventually, Sam's weight was so excessive that he felt more stress, which in turn caused him to eat more. In Chapter 14 we will present a method for Sam to develop his cognitive control.

Think about the triggers and habitual responses that are common in our society:

Conflict →	Drinking alcohol
Stress →	Smoking cigarettes
Rude behavior by another driver →	Road rage
Insult →	Retaliation
Unhappiness →	Drugs

Whether we're talking about routines (such as what TV shows we watch) or impulses (late-night snacking), these habits are triggered by something. These triggers are often unavoidable, so the only healthy response is to control them through activation of the prefrontal cortex.

Developing Controlled Responses

Our large prefrontal cortex is what separates us from other animals who live solely by routine and impulse. You must overcome and control impulses that need not be automatic. Such controlled responses can be operationalized by education and focused practice until your brain, in effect, rewires itself. Neuroscience has taught us that you can make brain changes, just as you upgrade your computer. Understanding the process is important, so identification of triggers that initiate unhealthy habits must be replaced with healthier responses.[226]

To understand that point, we must face up to the truth that we often miss. Remember the old axiom, "What a fish is least aware of is water." The truth is that we live in a human-made world we have invented; look at other animals then look at us. Most of what we do, use, and pay attention to is of our own creation. In a very literal sense, the human world is an unnatural world, an artificial world. This is not a criticism but a fact. But the human organism itself, including the brain and the nervous system, has changed little over the ages. We know we can never put a moratorium on technological invention, so if we are to hope for a viable change, we must start exploring ways to reinvent and evolve human nature. We must utilize psychology with the marvelous ingenuity and energy that we have devoted to technology and neuroscience findings. We must recognize and promote change that will produce another step in the evolution of our brain.

Healthy behaviors can be based on actions that we reflect upon and decide to control. Your automatic responses should not rule you. For example, you can plan your desired behaviors, how much you want to eat, to drink, to exercise, and plan accordingly. By focusing on habits that you want to control, you can resist yielding to automatic responses by making controlled responses that you have planned.

Examples of successful transfer of automatic responses to controlled ones are abundant. Overeaters who transition to healthy eating habits and recovering alcoholics provide models. Dr. Jonathan Page has been retraining police officers who, under stress, feel threatened and automatically respond to threatening situations by overreacting and resorting to violence.[227] Dr. Page's program will be explained in Chapter 14.

During the last decade, scientific writers have introduced popular audiences to theories, both sophisticated and simplistic, regarding the functioning of the brain. Malcolm Gladwell wrote a best-selling book in 2005 that introduced us to the power of intuition.[228] Gladwell points out that seemingly intuitive responses are actually a matter of a trained brain processing input at a high speed. Intuition is hardly foolproof, however. President Harding was elected mainly because he looked like a strong and decisive leader. Harding's presidency proved looks can be deceiving.

Self-regulation requires great effort, training and determination. Genuine change requires an understanding of the cravings that drive our behaviors. Charles Duhigg, a business reporter, explored habit change in his best-selling book *The Power of Habit*. He identifies a "habit loop" consisting of a cue (trigger), a routine, and a reward. He believes that the routine must be replaced. "If we keep the same cue and the same reward, a new routine can be inserted."[229] Reinforcement by a friend or a support group greatly facilitates change as demonstrated by Alcoholics Anonymous. Duhigg points out the possibilities:

> We know that change can happen. Alcoholics can stop drinking. Smokers can quit puffing. Perennial losers can become champions. You can stop biting your nails or snacking at work, yelling at your kids, staying up all night, or worrying over small concerns.[230]

Think about your typical day: You **awake to an alarm clock** that was set using your reflective process (what time do I need to get up in terms of my planned schedule); **brush your teeth** in a controlled way (how long, which toothpaste, how thorough); **choose and prepare breakfast** (content, portion size, and mode of preparation). These repeated controlled processes may seem automatic but are based on prior reflection and are self-regulated. We tend to give little thought to such daily routines, but the consequences of all this personal behavior still play a major role in our health and well-being.

Educator Barbara Given has aptly pointed out:

> Although the reflective learning system is the last to develop biologically, it is the most humane of all learning systems, acting as the brain's chief executive officer to integrate the organ's oldest and newest parts into a cohesive whole. Without explicit instruction in self-monitoring and performance analysis, however, this system can go dreadfully underdeveloped.[231]

We believe that many societal problems are the result of responding automatically to the reptilian brain rather than developing and using reflective capabilities and practicing self-regulation. The first step to developing controlled responses is to select your best options.

Humans continue to evolve, physically as well as mentally. For example, the changes in human height in the past 100 years have been extraordinary. We also know that focused educational efforts can change our brains and our behaviors. We propose establishing such a focus in our schools on **healthy communication**. We now know enough about the brain to build an educational framework based on neuroscience research to be a viable model of teaching and learning.[232]

Fear: The Illusion of Powerlessness

Throughout the 20th Century Americans had the illusion of safety from foreign enemies. On September 11, 2001 that illusion was shattered and replaced with another—that we are now vulnerable and our power is limited.

The human-made violence and damage to human life are the essence of every daily newspaper and media broadcast. Each day brings its own threats, emanating from international terrorists, domestic terrorists, violent criminals, scam artists, and political actions. Add to that: automobile accidents, unexpected health problems, fear of infection, plane accidents, fires, floods and explosions. All these events and possibilities can lead to greater personal stress and threats to your health and well-being. Should you live in fear? What can you do? Is everything going to be all right?[233]

The simple answer to the last question is "NO!" Everything is never all right. But with the same confidence, we predict that you will be all right. In all likelihood, you are not going to be the victim of a terrorist attack, killed in a plane crash or die of a falling object from the sky. Nor will you be shot in a drive-by crime. As President FDR told us, "The only thing we have to fear, is fear itself."

Like other aspects of our lives and health, fear can be seen as a continuum with unhealthy fear at one end and healthy fear at the other. Healthy fear keeps you alert, motivated and safer, such as when you are using a ladder or standing on a narrow ledge. Fear of disease may encourage you toward a healthier lifestyle as when you quit smoking or begin exercising. But when you are fearful of things that are unlikely to harm you, or overly fearful of something you cannot avoid, such as aging, then your fear is unhealthy and makes you unhappy and unmotivated.

We have cited many potential fears: death, terrorism, failure, being separated from people we love, rejection and loss of income. According to the teaching of Buddha, many such fears can be identified as "delusions," distorted ways of looking at the world and ourselves. Buddha's teachings are designed to overcome delusions, which are the source of our fears, by gaining control of our mind.[234]

Fear and stress affect the body in a similar fashion. The lungs expand so that more oxygen is available to the bloodstream and blood pressure rises as it is directed to the brain. This increased blood pressure, rapid heart rate, and high levels of cortisol weaken the body's organs if the fear persists for a long period. Putting your body in a constant state of agitation can wear down your heart, kill cells in the brain, and predispose you to diseases. People who want to live longer need to avoid unnecessary worrying about things they can't control.

With close friends, discuss the major things that you fear. Are these fears healthy or unhealthy? Fear and stress can be damaging to our health. Discuss the topics worthy of fear and those things that cannot be controlled.

Change is inevitable in your life and throughout society. To the extent that you have influence and input into the decisions that will guide the future of your nation and world, you must be an active participant. An educated, intelligent, and empowered society must assert values, rationality, and compassion in our decision making.

We have assertively presented five societal goals that we believe will help maintain a healthier world. We also encourage greater emphasis on education that utilizes neuroscience for developing greater use of controlled behaviors to replace automatic ones. Our habits and triggers must change to controlled responses if we are to achieve better health.

Chapter 13 - A Lifelong Plan for Healthy Communication

Your future will be determined by the choices you make today. What you decide and plan for today will shape who you become as an individual, and how you will impact your family and your nation. As demonstrated throughout the book, small changes can forge pathways to significant results. In this chapter, we present a plan for promoting healthy communication throughout a lifetime. You will discover that you already employ some of the behaviors and strategies. Others you will want to adapt or personalize to meet your own needs.

Social Roles in the Healthy Family

Social roles make life with others possible by providing predictability and stability. Sociologists state that social roles are necessary ways for people to divide the labor of society and establish a framework for interacting with others. The ability to master a variety of roles throughout life is a decided asset for healthy people because it facilitates easy interactions with others. You want to know what is expected of others similar to you in profession, age, and gender. This information provides a basis to predict and control reactions. From earliest childhood, everyone emulates the behavior of people who function as exemplars and role models. You learn much from your parents or caretakers including how to be a parent yourself. The experiences of being "in" and "of" a family are essential to a child's sense of identity in addition to fulfilling the needs for security and feeling loved.

Conversely, these roles can be an obvious or unrecognized source of stress and demoralization, literally making people sick. Roles can limit your identity, create stressful expectations, and block efforts to be authentic and empowered. Authority figures may threaten withdrawal of love and friendship if roles are disregarded. Parents, teachers, and authoritative adults have been permitted to impose strict, predictable rules for roles such as gender and social status.

In the past, assigned social roles automatically entitled certain individuals to privileges and rights, while denying them to others. The female roles, historically, condemned women to fewer educational opportunities, few job options, lower occupational status and pay, and, often, the exclusive responsibility for raising children. Men were often locked into a role defined in terms of strength, non-emotional behavior, and bread winning.

The traditional family roles followed stereotypical patterns that proved too limiting, resulting in problems for the individual and relationships. Stereotypical family expectations may be detrimental to your health. For example, filling the traditional mother role requires behavior of a woman that sometimes contributes to her emotional and physical detriment. The traditional father's role calls on him to be a "good provider" and lead a life of upward mobility, which created considerable stress. Matters become confusing when the same behaviors praised in men are criticized in women. A person needs to have the freedom and responsibility to do the best with their own needs/wishes and capabilities. Everyone should be able to choose to conform to roles, refuse them, or modify them in creative ways.

You have experienced in your lifetime an evolution of greater freedom for people to choose and define their identities and roles. While remnants of the stereotypic limitations linger, our society, fortunately, has evolved to far greater freedoms. Many fathers now take an active part in child rearing and household management, while mothers may choose to work in demanding jobs and manage the family budget. In an atmosphere of healthy communication, these issues can be openly addressed and resolved to the mutual satisfaction of both spouses and partners.

What has been your family history in terms of gender roles? Compare your parents' division of labor with your own relationships. Do you feel an equitable adjustment has been made?

As you expand your roles to include behavior and responsibilities not traditionally defined, you must recognize the psychological dangers of failure to redefine conflicting expectations. For example, the working mother who insists on being the only one to complete domestic duties puts herself under the stress of being a "superwoman" when duties at work and at home arise simultaneously. She may define herself as a bad mother or wife if she chooses her work obligation, or she may suffer poor work reviews by prioritizing her home obligation. The stay-at-home father who doesn't redefine his role may perceive himself as "less than a man" because he's not the breadwinner. All too frequently, "having it all" means attempting to "do it all." Role redefinition is more than a mere indulgence; it involves redefining values and redistributing duties with others.

Promoting Healthy Communication in the Family

When people choose a long-term partnership, each individual brings to the relationship different life experiences, values and priorities, personal habits, and other profound differences in taste, money, and time management. Each partner will have an initial learning curve.

Often partners find that this initial learning stage is mutually rewarding because each becomes better in touch with their own feelings and values as well as their partner's. Under the right circumstances, the communication becomes more open and involves more mutual listening. Communication based on genuine feelings of love, caring, and a goal of greater connectedness provides a foundation for a fulfilling life-long partnership. This healthy pattern of communication provides greater mutual trust, personal growth, and shared interests. As partners communicate more openly and deeply, they discover and develop more interests, values, and ambitions to explore together.

In his model depicting relational growth, Mark Knapp[235] identified a time after partners have melded into a couple when they must reassert themselves as individuals. Partners might come to need more living space for outside interests, time alone, and other friendships. Accepting one's own needs and a partner's needs to enrich life separately in no way contradicts the search for a wider and deeper mutual life within the relationship.

As we couple, personal problems become shared problems. Issues of health and wellness can be mutually explored and planned. Physical exercise can be reinforced by doing it together. Whether working out or going dancing, a mutually enjoyable activity can boost both physical and mental health while also enhancing the relationship. Mutual caring can help protect health by promoting good diets, sufficient sleep, and support for healthy habits.

A need to have "alone" time is important, too. Both partners need to incorporate time for themselves – whether for reading, exercise, naps, meditation, bubble baths, or time to practice a hobby or art. Partners can provide this time for each other by minding children alone for an hour or so. One couple we know did this each Saturday morning as one partner took their daughter for "just us time" while the other partner had "just me time." At another time in the week, it was the reverse.

A Healthy Communication Session Plan

As children are added to your family, we suggest establishing a set time each week for a *healthy communication session* as a tool in guaranteeing healthy communication throughout the life of an intimate relationship. A private comfortable space should be used that can be protected from phone calls and other media interruptions. Two hours is ideal. During this time, focus is on the participants, starting with the two partners and expanding as children or other family members are added. No one is too young or too old.

The ground rules are simple. Everyone here is valued, loved, and will be treated with unconditional personal regard. You will be exclusively focused on one another for the time allotted. You are protected by confidentiality and will give priority to the here-and-now; that is, what you are currently thinking and feeling. In keeping with these guidelines, we recommend the following commitments:

1. You will be honest and truthful with one another. You will do your best to understand one another, repeating your understandings until all parties are satisfied.

2. Confidentiality will be respected and maintained. Information shared at this time will not become a matter for teasing nor shaming. The only reason for disclosing beyond the confines of this safe place is if there is reason to believe that someone will suffer harm by maintaining secrecy. Any sharing of secrets will be to agents of assistance such as parents, doctors, counselors, or law enforcement officials.

3. You will listen with empathy and caring.

4. You will empower each other to share thoughts and feelings without sanctions or defensiveness. Explorations are welcome.

These times are easy to build into the beginning of a relationship as you are highly motivated to get to know and understand each other. They are equally important and enjoyable in all stages of a relationship and should be continued. People and relationships are a constant process; you will want to stay abreast of the changes. If together time starts to feel burdensome or obligatory, that in itself becomes a topic for discussion. As time marches on, these "us times" become more difficult to hold as a high priority without intentional effort. A couple in a long-term relationship encounters outside time demands, jobs, aging parents, and other obligations. Dates, "dates at home," pillow talk, and times set aside are perfect occasions to explore each other's lives, views, feelings, and attitudes. All offer opportunities to reveal and explore subjects and emotions that can otherwise be overlooked or sublimated. Tending to issues as they arise makes it easier to maintain a good relationship and much easier than repairing a damaged one later.

Such time is especially difficult to set aside when a child is born. Parents are busy accommodating the needs of the newest member of their family while meeting other obligations. For many parents, getting enough sleep becomes one of the highest priorities. Individual and relational needs are sacrificed. Times with each other are important, but terribly difficult to schedule with a newborn. Exhaustion, disruption, and changing professional demands are stressful and can sometimes put partnerships in jeopardy. Young mothers can have postpartum depression; young fathers can feel overlooked and underappreciated. Together-time provides opportunities to explore these feelings and seek remedies. Timely discussions can circumvent "festering" resentments or issues.

Babies, toddlers, and young children are obviously unable to sit through two hours of talking. Early sessions can be improvised as needed. Good questions to begin with might be "What happened?" or "How do you feel?" Helping young children identify emotions and indicating that their experiences are important allows them to share now and prepares them to happily continue as they get older. Creating early focused times with children, even if it is a reading time or playing games, makes the child feel loved and included and willing to share. They also prepare children to identify and express their feelings.

Some families, as problems arise, are able to interrupt their schedule and insert "us" time as it is needed. Many families caught up in the hustle and bustle of daily living must set aside a designated time to ensure that it will happen each week.

If you are instituting these times as an already established family, the sessions may seem awkward at first. You must be tolerant and patient as you set up the right communication environment. A period of silence does not mean that no thinking is taking place. In this leaderless format, it is important for parents to resist being directive, authoritarian, or punitive. All participants must commit to "being tuned in" at all times. Personal questions are welcomed: "What are you feeling right now?" "How do you respond to my choice of...?" "What concerns you now?" "Why are you worrying?"

Introducing children to this session should be done with sensitivity. Give them opportunities for involvement at an early age. Ideally, these sessions will grow naturally out of loving parents meeting the special requirements of infants. You may need to get creative as children grow and fuller schedules evolve, but be diligent and you'll experience rewards. Discussions within the family can empower children. For example: when a child comes home angry about another child's behavior, it would make sense to ask your child for a preferred outcome to the situation. Point out to your child that another child's behavior is not under her control but her own behavior is. An exploration of her immediate emotions affirms the child's experience. Follow that with a discussion of reasonable responses most likely to lead to the desired outcome. Your children will discover their own ability to be disciplined even when others are being unreasonable, rude, or just plain mean. This discussion of alternative responses in spontaneous "us" time actually helps your child become empowered by exploring and practicing responses for the future.

The earliest foundations for "us time" begin while cuddling and feeding infants and changing their diapers, teaching toddlers to identify emotions as they feel them ("Are you happy? Oh, you are sad,"), and behaving empathically ("Oh look, poor kitty is hungry. Let's feed her,") and kindly ("Be gentle with the puppy,") as a behavior model. Reading books to toddlers and young children provides many opportunities for discussion, and lays a verbal foundation for longer discussions later. Early foundations of listening can be set when the nonverbal toddler expresses desires ("Oh, you want mommy to hold you?") and when you respond to monosyllabic words. If you want your children to talk to you in their teen years, show them you care about what they have to "say" from birth and that you'll help them meet their goals and desires.

Family activities (long drives together, vacations, game nights, camping trips, etc.) can provide opportunities for "us" times so long as there is time for focused discussion and the activity does not interfere with connecting with each other. The goals of family time are consistent; to build bonds between family members, to facilitate the healthy development of each family member, to update our impressions of each member, to support one another, and to keep the family and its members functional. It is natural for the manifestation of family times to change according to the needs of growing individuals, but family times should not be abandoned.

You will get feedback from your family members through their attention, focus, and, hopefully, feelings of love. Be patient, and don't give up too soon if you don't feel you are getting instant rewards. Start toddlers with brief sessions and extend the time as vocabulary and attention spans increase. We predict that a family will learn to value and welcome this opportunity.

Plan the timing of each session for a designated time that will have priority on your schedule and everyone's full attention. Preserving and protecting this time-frame may present a challenge. Perhaps your family meets Tuesday evening from 7:30-10:00 pm, or Sunday from 2:00-4:00 pm; house guests can be informed that the family time is private, and they can have free time for themselves. Telephone calls will not be answered except in case of emergency, and no television or social media is allowed. Neuroscientists Adam Gazzaley and Larry D. Rosen have found that having cell phones within view creates enough distraction that our thinking is slowed, and we have greater trouble focusing on each other.[236]

The family dinner hour used to allow family members time to keep up with one another. Unfortunately, families often find no time to share meals today and intimate, meaningful communication occurs irregularly. Consequently, the focused time together, suggested here, will become a highlight on your schedule and greatly enrich the lives of each family member.

Parenting and Infancy

Honest expressions of love, caring, and commitment are important in all phases of life, but crucial at the beginning. Newborns need a great deal of assistance in acclimating to the new world. Parents can and should be the face of the child's developing world. They are the source of comfort and security, and dispellers of pain and fear. In every waking hour, the child learns about him/herself from parents and their touch, love, and responsiveness. Numerous studies have concluded that babies left without sufficient attention –who are not spoken to, held, comforted, or shown love – grow to feel helpless and without a sense of well-being.

The parents' goal should be to raise reasonable, socialized children who have strong self-esteem. Patterns of communication need to be established that will promote a loving relationship that provides the child with basic needs, safety, and a sense of shared understandings, with reasonable expectations and little conflict. Psychologists Matthew McKay and Patrick Fanning have cited four ways parents can contribute to a child's developing self-esteem.

1. Recognize your child's unique abilities and talents. Periodically think about qualities or abilities that are truly strengths or talents, and reinforce the behavior by recognizing, praising and rewarding it, making it more likely the child will want to do it again. Monitor your child's determination to achieve, as well as their happiness and coordination.

2. Understand the child's behavior in the context of who they are. Validate life-enhancing needs and feelings. Avoid judgmental "shoulds." Don't utilize guilt, withholding of affection, or anger as negative enforcers.

3. See children accurately and focus negatively on behavior that needs to be changed: behaviors that are harmful to them, behaviors that isolate them socially, or are disruptive to the family. Try to determine what need is being addressed by the behavior. Perhaps the need can be met in a more appropriate way.

4. If parents unconditionally accept all of their child, she can accept herself. The acceptance is the cornerstone of good self-esteem. Children who feel they are really seen and understood by their parents can afford to be authentic. Such children don't have to hide parts of themselves for fear of being rejected.[237]

We have previously introduced the "Roots of Empathy" program designed to nurture and develop empathy and social literacy in all children. The program begins in kindergarten and extends through middle school. It is now used in about a dozen countries and has demonstrated effectiveness in its outcomes.[238] The premise of the program is that if children are able to take the perspective of the "other," they will notice and appreciate commonalities, and be less likely to exaggerate differences that lead to conflict, dislike, and even violence.

A young mother and her baby, (in this case five-month-old Tomas) make reoccurring visits to a classroom of kindergartners who will follow Tomas's progress throughout their elementary years. A green blanket is placed on the floor, and the children arrange themselves cross-legged on the floor around the blanket. The baby is clearly excited as his mother moves around the students giving each the opportunity to greet baby Tomas. Tomas is placed on his tummy on the blanket and a toy that he likes is also placed on the floor. The children observe Tomas's eyes and face as they sing a jingle and offer words of encouragement, such as "Way to go, Tomas," as he locates the toy. Tomas's mother is impressed by the interest the children take in her son's development and moved by their obvious excitement at every new thing Tomas learns.

The children will spend time with the instructor in the week prior to Tomas's visit, predicting what he will be able to do. They will spend time in the week after Tomas's visit exploring what they learned and connecting it to their own development and feelings, and then the big leap – gaining an understanding of their classmates' feelings.

Tomas and his mother will visit this class every month for the school year. The children will be coached by the instructor to observe the parent-child relationship, the baby's development, the baby's temperament, their own temperament, and that of their classmates. They will learn about infant safety and issues that have an impact on their own well-being and security. They will learn how an understanding of temperament and gaining insights into their own emotions, and those of others, leads to empathy and builds rich human relationships.[239]

While we encourage the inclusion of the "Roots of Empathy" program in schools, some of the experiences can also be utilized within families in their healthy communication sessions.

Family sessions can also serve as age appropriate check-points for good health practices – diet, exercise, sleep, teeth brushing, and emotional issues. Early foundations can be laid for talking candidly as children mature and need to learn about issues related to their development. Those early discussions lay foundations for discussions to follow; puberty, body odor, and safe sex. Difficult discussions may also include death, loss of loved ones, and changes in parental marital status. Discussions invite and explain change and provide emotional support for children and partners as we navigate our life paths.

Adolescence and Early Adulthood

Physical health becomes a necessary topic for candid discussion during the period of adolescence. Weight control and fitness are always important for good general health and self-esteem. Maintaining a healthy diet and sufficient exercise (at least an hour a day for young people) are whole-family issues. Care must be taken to protect teenagers from excessive emphasis on appearance that can trigger unhealthy body-image issues.

Dr. Michael Weitzman, Professor of Pediatrics and Psychiatry at NYU says, "Teens are moody. There's no way around that." Mood swings are normal and expected, but if moodiness persists for over a week and seems to damage performance at school or friendships, "this behavior should raise a red flag for parents that something might be wrong."[240] Middle school and high school are stressful, and with this increased stress comes the risk of depression and experimentation with drugs, alcohol, and/or sex. Parental communication is needed to catch early signs of problems that may be arising at school or with friends.

Young adulthood brings about necessary life changes and, often, accompanying stress; finishing education, entering the workplace, entering serious new relationships, and some degree of physical separation from the parents. Hopefully, healthy communication sessions continue, along with attitudes and skills for maintaining authentic, empathic communication. These young adults are likely to discuss their career paths with their families and ask for guidance when making decisions about their careers. Grown children are likely to visit the family and renew the bonds and mutual sharing.

Young adults should establish relationships with a physician and other health providers and be mindful of their mental states. This transitional time in their lives might produce increased anxiety and stress. It is important to seek help from mental health providers if needed. The National Institute of Mental Health can be consulted on line or through a family physician.

Living Life Single

Most individuals will live at least part of their adult lives independently. According to the United States Census, 47 percent of all Americans over the age of eighteen are single. On average, Americans spend more than half of their adulthood single. There are biases in our society that suggests single existence is of a lower quality than having a partner, but there is good reason to challenge such an assumption. About half of all American marriages end in divorce, and second and third marriages have an even greater chance of failure. The body of work by Bella DePaulo, a Harvard Ph.D., suggests that single lives can be healthy lives, and cultural bias may be the reason the single life has been perceived as unhealthy. For most of us, the healthy psychological state associated with personal success is determined by a combination of happiness, achievement, significance, and legacy. While you may occasionally short one or more of these components for another, you are seldom satisfied with a life that does not maintain all components in balance. Although there is some evidence (the significance of which DePaulo questions) that married individuals live longer than singles, there is also evidence that single life may be healthier than married life. DePaulo identifies research indicating that singles exercise more and gain less weight. Single men suffer less frequently from heart attacks.[241] Singles tend to spend their healthy communication time with a larger network of friends and family than those in partnerships. Singles spend more time caring for parents and they maintain closer relationships with their siblings.[242]

Some singles consider themselves "temporarily single." Others are content in their single life styles without seeking to change their status. It is interesting to note that greater self-sufficiency inspires positive feelings in singles but inspires negative feelings in those who are or have been married.[243]

DePaulo points out that home life arrangements are changing. While nuclear family and communal life styles are declining, all other arrangements are increasing. Children are living with their parents longer or returning to the nest. Divorced parents raise their children successfully. Single parents are creating healthy homes for their children. Like-minded single people who want to have children are deciding to have and raise children together without becoming romantically involved. Single moms are combining households without romantic or legal attachments.[244] Single people can maintain healthy connections and lifestyles and, when they desire, they may choose unconventional methods of creating families.

Late 20's to 40's

This is the stage of life when many are completing professional school educations, developing their careers, entering marriage, and possibly starting families of their own. The healthy communication sessions that once were part of your childhood are now hopefully part of your current relationships with your partner and children. It is very important that you have developed a relationship with a physician by this time in your life as there are necessary medical screenings that should be done to promote wellness.

Middle to Old Age

Maturity! You are fortunate if you have remained healthy through a long life. You must be doing some things right or, at least, the necessary things. Your quest for increased self-understanding and lifelong self-improvement has been a challenging journey. Benjamin Franklin reportedly said: "We get old too soon, and wise too late." Based on the values and aspirations we have articulated in this book, we believe that the true yardstick of a mature person is best viewed from the perspective of human relations. The healthy mature person demonstrates the following:

- confidence in his/her ability to relate to others. Such a person demonstrates trust of self and the capacity to trust others.
- empathy and non-possessive acceptance of others. This person is a good listener and lets others know that she/he cares.
- communicates in a congruent manner. Values, feelings, and opinions are expressed in a way that lets you know what he/she really thinks.
- adaptable and changes behavior without tensions or confusion if he/she chooses to change. This person is attentive to feedback to find new ways of relating to and working with others.
- assumes responsibility for their physical, emotional, and spiritual needs.
- knows him/herself, enjoys fulfilling relationships and participates in local/state/national governance through knowledgeable votes and assertive expression.

Thus, healthy, mature people demonstrate a mastery of the process of relating to others and changing behaviors as necessary or appropriate. They have brought their *perceived self* and *ideal self*-closer together and have a high level of self-acceptance and well-being.

A lifetime of healthy eating and appropriate exercise pays off in later adulthood.

These people have a lower risk of disease, depression, and chronic pain, and are less vulnerable to dementia than their less fit peers. A study found that adults aged seventy to seventy-nine who maintained their mental acuity had several things in common: they exercised at least once a week, did not smoke, had at least a high school education, and were socially active. According to experts on aging, that last point is crucial. "Social connection – with friends or family or within the community – helps keep a mind healthy. Likewise, isolation can be a mark of decline."

Elders with Issues

Personal Problems—As we age, we will encounter health problems, some expected and others without warning. The 2020 pandemic was such an event. To the extent possible, you need to plan your reactions to emergencies. Your backup safety plan should include:

- Gather the names and addresses of temporary safe locations that provide help you may require such as hospitals, basements, shelters, and health facilities.
- Keep a week's supply of food and water available and accessible.
- Have available contact information for agencies or companies responsible for power and for local emergency services such as fire, police, and medical technicians, as well as friends or neighbors you can count on in an emergency.
- Learn the facts and decide in advance. Does any agency in your community monitor a list of people who should be helped first in the event of a disaster? If the phone service is not working, how can you contact emergency management?

If you are in an assisted living situation, chances are high that you'll experience a problem at some point with the care you receive or the person or agency providing the care or services. If the problem involves abuse, violence, neglect, theft, or other serious wrong-doing, call 911 and/or Adult Protective Services immediately for help. The close proximity of residents and absence of appropriate sanitization have led to disproportionate numbers of coronavirus cases and deaths.

For procedural or non-emergency problems, follow these guidelines:

- Communicate clearly what your needs are and what you are asking of the person or agency. Confirm their understanding about what you want. Repeat as often as necessary to achieve mutual understanding.
- Address a problem as soon as possible. Get others involved who can help you as soon as you are not in danger. Write down details and save a record of events such as the dates you talked about the problem and with whom as well as what was agreed to be done to correct the problem.

- Listen and reflect. Have clarity on what caused the problem and what is needed to prevent a recurrence.
- Take appropriate action. If the problem concerns a caregiver, a replacement may be called for. Your well-being is the most important consideration. If you cannot act on your own behalf, ask someone to do it for you. You may have to put something in writing for your representative to talk freely with your caregivers without breaking privacy rules.

If you choose to stay in your own home and maintain your independence, consider the following modifications: using computers and related technological equipment such as "Echo," "Siri," or "Alexa" which respond to voice commands and can turn off and on lights and appliances; setting electronic medication reminders and dispensers; and employing assistive devices including ramps, chair lifts, and grab bars to make your home safer and more accessible.

As you make decisions on remaining at home or choosing an assisted living facility, talk with your doctor and the local agency on aging. Strongly consider having a lawyer help you prepare a "living will" so that your own preferences will be followed if needed.

Dr. Jen's Rx

For...

Address...

R_X Date:............................

Our brains don't shrink with age because we actually generate thousands of new neurons every day through a process called neurogenesis. Lack of sleep and stress slow the process down, while vigorous exercise speeds it up. People tend to think more slowly as they age, but the ability to "see the big picture" improves with age.

Refills NA 1 2 3 4 5

Signature...

Healthy Communication Outside the Home

To this point, we have discussed primarily the private, intimate communication with family and close friends. Healthy communication also functions outside of the home in such sites as the workplace or in organizations to which you belong. Large bureaucratic organizations have long been criticized for their inhumanity and impersonality. Universities, as well as commercial organizations, have been guilty of reducing people to numbers and automatons, and promoting conformity in behavior, while producing elevated levels of stress and causing related health problems discussed in earlier chapters. Bureaucracy tends to define people by their position held to allow for easy replacement without concern for feelings.

For an organization to be truly healthy, we believe the following conditions are requisite:

- *Change is expected.* To the extent that rigidity and conformity are the rule, individual interpersonal growth is handicapped. Reverence for tradition has some merit, but is debilitating if that tradition does not include exploration and innovation.

- *Feedback is used.* Without the use of healthy communication to provide a reflection of how you are perceived by others, awareness of a needed behavior change is diminished. Feedback can motivate change, indicate type of change needed, and help one to evaluate attempts to achieve new behaviors.

- *Members are committed to each other.* When interpersonal commitment is present, a supportive climate assists members in explorative, innovative efforts. Members may not easily produce desired changes, but supported attempts make positive changes more likely. Likewise, a member has the right to choose not to change. The interpersonal demand should be only that feedback be accepted, and implied change be considered. Tolerance for individual differences will be given as much respect as adherence to patterns usually thought to be pleasing. In essence, a healthy person can tolerate individual differences in a climate where her needs are considered by others, and her own individual peculiarities are tolerated.

- *Decision making is shared.* Those who are affected by a decision have some voice in its making. This does not mean that every decision is made by a committee. Rather, the thinking and desires of those persons affected by the decision will be explored, respected, and considered. In many cases they will be given a vote; in all cases they will have a voice. As this opportunity is extended, more assume responsibility, grow in self-image and in the esteem of others. Growth, development, and maturity are thus related.

- *Personal growth is encouraged.* Leaders in the organization provide training and learning experiences for their subordinates. As additional responsibility is assumed and successfully shouldered, persons are rewarded. Within the organization is a positive feeling that there is the opportunity for advancement, growth, and development. Instead of griping about their situation, people are encouraged to do something about it, to take on greater responsibilities, to share in the task of improving their environment, and to become more capable individuals – both in terms of professional or occupational expertise and interpersonal relating.

- In a healthy organization where team spirit prevails, members can share even polemic information. They voice honestly their disagreements. Problems are openly addressed and resolved by an agreed upon process. Since the group is trained in empathic listening and shared problem solving and compromise, a mutually acceptable resolution is usually found.

Remember that criticism of behavior and identification of consequences is preferred over applying judgmental labels. They provide your target with actions to take and insight regarding the value of a desired action. Note the difference between saying "You're a slob! Clean up"! And "We distract each other from work when our (shared) office is cluttered with tools and supplies. If we put away tools, supplies and projects as they are completed, our mutual productivity would increase."

In addition to the attitudinal and behavioral considerations, skills for communicating in the work environment are important. Two excellent books are available that provide useful information. *Communicating with Results* is already in the 11th edition (2018) and covers every aspect of the communication process in the business organization. *Business and Professional Communication: Keys for Workplace Excellence* (2019) puts its emphasis on business writing and professional

In your work life, have your workplaces been as functional as possible? How would you characterize the communication climate? Is there anything you could have done to improve your work climate? What have been your leadership opportunities and experiences with those above you?

presentation.[245] Both books are authoritative and accessible, and are available on Amazon.

An excellent guide to effective strategic leadership for the modern organization is the *U. S. Army Leadership Field Manual*. Developed over decades, this field manual is based on sound psychological research and psychiatric theory and articulates the core requisites for military leaders to do their jobs effectively.[246] Foremost among the crucial qualities fundamental for leadership is trust. As the Manual states: "leaders shape the ethical climate of their organization while developing the trust and relationships that enable proper leadership."[247] Chicago psychiatrist Prudence Gourguechon has suggested that the Army Manual provides an excellent source for evaluating all leaders of great responsibility. She states: "A leader who is deficient in the capacity for trust makes little effort to support others, may be isolated and aloof, may be apathetic about discrimination, allows distrustful behaviors to persist among team members, makes unrealistic promises, and focuses on self-promotion."[248] All leaders must be trustworthy.

Discipline and self-control are crucial to effective leadership according to the *Manual*. Effective leaders do not have emotional outbursts or act impulsively; they think reflectively before jumping into action. We suggest that proper training has prepared the leader with cognitive control for emergencies. Control is required to keep the leader from saying or doing whatever comes to mind.

Judgment and critical thinking require a leader who "seeks to obtain the most thorough and accurate understanding possible."[249] He/she anticipates "first, second, and third consequences of multiple courses of action."[250] Note the requirement for process thinking and being able to predict accurately the consequences of actions.

Self-awareness requires that leaders "know themselves, including their traits, feelings and behaviors. They employ self-understanding and recognize their effect on others." The absence of self-understanding may result in tendencies to blame others for problems and ignore feedback.

The final essential attribute cited as critical for effective Army leadership is, unsurprisingly, empathy. The good leader must "demonstrate an understanding of another person's point of view and identifies with others' feelings and emotions."[251] Without empathy, you can't perceive and respond to another's emotional distress.

The qualities reflective of healthy communication are guidelines for all effective leadership. They show maturity and a concern for the health of all involved.

Organizations must recognize the importance of change, feedback, and shared decision-making to promote a healthy work environment. Finally, our elected leaders should follow the guidelines of the *U. S. Army Leadership Field Manual*. If we cannot trust our leaders and know that they are disciplined, authentic, and empathetic, then we will never know who they are truly serving.

Dr. Jen's Rx

For...

Address...

Rx   Date:.........................

*The saddest fact in life is not that people
have to suffer in order to grow, but that
many people persist in suffering without
growing.*

Refills NA 1 2 3 4 5

Signature...

We have made our case for a change in direction for our country. In the previous chapters we have presented a rationale in three major areas – authenticity, empathy, and empowerment. Unfortunately, our country has been often moving in the wrong direction, heading toward unhealthy outcomes.

We look forward to a different sort of country emerging from the pandemic.

Personal Reflection

In your work life, have your workplaces been as functional as possible? How would you characterize the communication climate? Is there anything you could do to improve your work climate? What have been your leadership opportunities and experiences in your job?

Chapter 14 - Developing Attitudes and Skills for Healthy Communication

The importance of utilizing healthy communication has been made clear. If you wish to understand yourself better, and are interested and willing to change your attitudes and communication behaviors to contribute to a healthier and happier future, this chapter provides a path to take. Our suggestions are based on our beliefs that people have the freedom and capacity to change themselves and their world. We will supply some resources and guidelines that can promote and operationalize self-change. Permanent self-change is based on a commitment to break away from the old, unhealthy ways of thinking and behaving and to create new patterns for a healthier life. First, you will determine which behaviors you need to change and then chart a personal plan for accomplishing the changes.

Healthy communicators are aware that they are continually in process – always changing. This awareness validates that they are alive, spontaneous, and willing to take risks. Feelings such as joy and sadness, likes and dislikes, are openly acknowledged and expressed. Complex, mixed, and even contradictory emotions are recognized and shared. Every day is experienced as an adventure where everything is possible, and anything can be tried. As far back as 500 BC the Greek philosopher Heraclitus asserted that "to live is to change." The world is changing in ways that a person cannot always control. Technology, the environment, and governmental policies seem to change frequently and often radically. Relationships can come and go, created by circumstances, such as moving to a new location. A person must be able to come to terms with the change and respond appropriately. The human brain permits us to make a reflective response instead of automatic ones.

Identifying Barriers to Healthy Communication

Psychological threats to the self are processed in the same fashion as physical threats, and your automatic responses to them are much the same as well. For example, when you feel that you are being treated impersonally, defense mechanisms automatically engage. The defensive individual is likely unaware that this choice is unhealthy and mitigates growth. A fundamental reason for defensive behavior appears to be the inability of many people to acknowledge differences – differences between perceptions and reality, and differences between our own perceptions and those of others. Psychologists have identified defense mechanisms that both impair growth and increase an unhealthy state of self-alienation. Among the common defensive mechanisms are the following:

- *Repression.* This pattern of response consists of actively excluding from one's self-awareness any thought, feeling, or suggestion that threatens one's self-image or the way one seeks to be perceived by others. If repressed too long, the emotions may erupt into hostile or violent actions.[252]

- *Rationalization.* This response is an explanation for one's behavior that serves to justify questionable conduct. Intentions are introduced that are at variance with others' perceived reality. Excuses such as "I was just kidding," or "I didn't mean anything by that," are thus provided for an objectionable behavior, but they are, of course, fake excuses.
- *Depersonalizing Others.* If someone views others as less than human, it becomes possible to mistreat them without feeling guilty. Such depersonalization makes possible acts of extreme violence.

Dr. Jen's Rx

For...

Address...

Rx   Date:.........................

After a day of appropriate exercise and diet, you are not just a day older. You are a day healthier!

Refills NA 1 2 3 4 5

Signature...

Defensive Behaviors

Note that, in the final analysis, such responses are used by people against perceived threats such as the threat of change or harm to one's personal view of the world. What healthy threat-reducing techniques are available to us?

The late Jack Gibb provided some significant answers through an eight-year study of interpersonal interactions. He was able to discern two communication styles – one defensive (threatening) and one supportive (healthy). We summarize and contrast Gibb's paired categories of perceived behavior in Table 14.1.[253] Defensiveness impedes healthy interactions. Defensive behavior of one person is likely to arouse defensiveness in the other. Conversely, the behaviors that are supportive promote reciprocity and healthy communication.

Table 14.1 Categories of Defensive and Supportive Behavior

SUPPORTIVE BEHAVIORS	DEFENSIVE BEHAVIORS
1. Description – nonjudgmental; to present feelings, perceptions, and a narrative that does not imply the receiver needs to change.	1. Evaluation – to pass judgment on another; to blame or praise; to question another's values, motives, and behavior.
2. Problem Orientation – a desire to collaborate in defining a mutual problem and finding a solution. Sharing information without a pre-conceived solution.	2. Control – to attempt to change an attitude or behavior of another; may involve coercion, persuasion, manipulation, or power to force change.
3. Spontaneity – being natural, straightforward, and honest; no hidden motives or deception.	3. Strategy – planning ways to use tricks and possible deception to get another to reach desired decision. May attempt to solicit false trust, as in a scam.
4. Empathy – showing respect for and identification with the other. Understanding and accepting their emotional values without trying to solve their problems.	4. Neutrality – to express a lack of concern for the welfare of another; remaining detached and clinical observer without emotions.
5. Equality – attracts little attention to ability, status, worth, or power. Planning is participative with mutual trust and respect.	5. Superiority – to emphasize one's own intellect, power, wealth and influence to create feelings of inadequacy in the other; absence of honest sharing.
6. Provisionalism – to problem solve rather than debate. To investigate and mutually share and critically access data.	6. Certainty – dogmatic, seems to know all the answers, needs no new information. Needing to be right and win the argument rather than solving a problem.

Distrust and Defensiveness

As we approach the end of our journey, we must be clear on the changes that need to be made. We believe the foremost problem in relating well to other people is distrust and its counter part, defensive interpersonal behavior. We have suggested that people need supportive feedback from valued others to achieve both a satisfying self-image and the basis for a continuing on-going relationship. When this need remains unmet, a feeling of anxiety is produced. The unresolved anger generates defensive tactics in relationships with others. These defensive behaviors are genuine and unconscious, and people usually perceive them accurately as signs of anxiety and fear. A direct personal attack is the most serious form of defensive stratagy and is likely viewed as overt, unprovoked agression.

Communication that Generates Defensiveness

Sometimes we find ourselves distrusting a person without knowing how it came about. Knowledge about communication behaviors that tend to increase distrust will help us forestall our trigger reactions of defensiveness. Investigation of such incidents has identified the following contributory conditions or causes of defensive behavior. We have selected examples from the recorded public appearances of former president Trump in his briefing responses to COVID-19.

1. Evaluation by expression, manner of speech, tone of voice, or verbal content, perceived by the receiver (listener) as criticism or judgment, will produce defensive behavior. Former president Trump showed judgmental behavior as he praised or blamed the governors in their responses to the coronavirus. Trump also displayed defensiveness in his threats, distortions, and use of needed resources as a reward. He cast blame widely and used fake data to justify the blame against many, including the Chinese, governors, past administrations, the democrats, the medical profession, and the World Health Organization.

2. Communication perceived by the recipient as an attempt to control him/her will produce defensiveness. Every briefing included Former President Trump's overt message of control. Every power at his disposal was utilized.

3. Stratagems that are perceived as clever devices produce defensiveness; partially hidden motives breed suspicion. Persons seen as "playing a game," feigning emotion, withholding information, or having private access to sources of data will stimulate defensive responses.

4. A lack of concern for the welfare of a person will heighten her/his need for defensiveness. Such "neutrality" may be necessary at times, but people strongly need to be perceived as valued persons. A clinically detached or impersonal manner (not caring) is usually feared and resented. We have already cited Trump's absence of empathy. There was never evidence of understanding or acceptance of the pain and risks felt by the citizens during the initial U.S. outbreak of COVID-19.

5. An attitude of superiority arouses defensive behavior; any behavior that reinforces the recipients's feelings of inadequacy is a source of disturbance. Trump often spoke of his "great brain and high intellect," and of being the most powerful man in the world and one of the richest. Trump compared himself to other U.S. presidents whom he said failed to measure up including Lincoln whom he said: "nearly lost the Civil War."[254]

6. Dogmatism is a well-known stimulus of defensive behavior; if you know something "for certain" it is wise to determine whether or not someone else wants to hear it from you and whether your answer

should be offered tentatively or with final certainty. Trump was the embodiment of certainty as described on Table 14.1. He presented himself as knowing all the answers and needing no additional information. He repeatedly said he knows more than the doctors. By needing to be right and winning every argument, the problems at hand went unaddressed.

Just as there is always some behavior you can change to promote your physical health, there is always some way to promote your communication health. Changing behaviors for the better takes planning. It doesn't happen by accident. Step-by-step planning involves having a clear idea of what you want, a plan for accomplishing the changes, and a way of evaluating your progress. A trusted partner may be necessary for feedback, encouragement, and validation. Such support has traditionally been offered by therapists but can be provided by any trusted knowledgeable person (spouses, religious leaders, sponsors, or close friends.)

Developing Healthy Communication through Greater Cognitive Control

Now would be a good time to review what we know about the brain. The automatic response system is the primitive, reptilian remnant of the survival instinct of all living creatures. The much later evolved reflective response system permits self-regulation as developed in the human cortex. (Refer to Figure 3.1). The brain has evolved and continues to do so. Many researchers advocate promoting human evolution through self-regulation and brain training. Your capability of developing controlled cognitive responses as a middle ground alternative between your automatic, and the much slower reflective system, offers you a methodology for such development.

The Brain and Goal-Setting

The frontal cortex is the core of the cognitive control network that literally controls billions of individual neurons. By using structural imaging to convert brain scans into "wiring diagrams," researchers have utilized control theory, a field previously used to study electrical systems, to provide an understanding of how you can achieve control over automatic processing. The prime usage of this understanding of how the brain controls its activities is directed at interventions in such medical conditions as schizophrenia, dementia or autism. Neuroscientists, however, are also able to visualize how the frontal cortex enables people to stay focused on one task or switch to a radically different one.[255] Akili Interactive Labs of Boston and Posit Science in San Francisco are conducting research regarding the use of video games as a way of rewiring neural connections of individuals with ADHD. Both companies are conducting controlled clinical trials in order to apply for FDA approval. Some conjecture that the treatment may one day prove as effective as drugs.[256] It has been shown that everyone can develop this kind of cognitive control through conscious effort and repetition.

Cognitive control is how the brain permits a person to choose a goal-serving behavior from competing options. Jonathan Cohen, Director of the Neuroscience Lab at Princeton University, believes that cognitive control underlies the capacity to make informed choices that "make us human," whether the choices are problem solving, language usage, planning, or reasoning.[257] Cohen goes on to connect cognitive control to "willpower," such as the delayed gratification in resisting a second serving of ice cream. In knowing the way your brain is disposed to behaving or misbehaving, in accordance to your goals, it's easier to get the results you're looking for, whether it's avoiding the temptation of chocolate cookies, or the pull of darkly ruminative thoughts.[258]

The brain has amazing capabilities. A person is able to combine any memory with all their life experiences and learnings from science, as well as hunches, guesses, dreams, and fantasies, to create new connections and, in concert with others, revolutionize society. Artists, creative people, and "geniuses" in all facets of life have such capacities to use their brains to advance the world with beauty, innovation, medical cures, and ways to solve significant problems.

Dr. Jonathan Page, a cognitive neuroscientist and co-founder of a private consulting company that trains police officers (whose work was introduced in Chapter 12), has developed a specific training program designed to wire the officers' brains to take fast and appropriate action based on a mental process of "cognitive command." He has built his program around three factors: *breathing, self-talk, and mental imagery.*[259]

Breathing as a Tool for Cognitive Control

Page first stresses that breathing helps to control the stress of the situation, keeps the heart rate down, and provides the necessary time to scan the surroundings for context, potential danger and threats, and mental review of known data. The goal is to "slow situations down," allowing the officer to be better able to make proper critical decisions and respond to the situation in the proper pre-planned manner. Responses to a variety of crises have been formulated and rehearsed before a crisis actually occurs.

Page provides a generic method of "tactical breathing": breathing in slowly through the nostrils, holding the breath for a few seconds, exhaling through the mouth, and waiting a few seconds before inhaling again. This practice is also common in sports; the great golfer Tom Watson reportedly said that he didn't learn to win under pressure until he learned to control his breathing.[260]

"Self-talk" as a Tool for Cognitive Control

The plan is set in motion by "self-talk" involving a code word to signal the best response. The code word triggers a pre-planned and pre-learned response. The word "finger," for instance, is used to train police officers not to shoot their guns prematurely. The code name has been practiced by tying the word to the motor behavioral response that best fits the circumstances. Repetitive conditioning builds muscle memory that helps guide the behavior subconsciously.[261]

Consider a situation where it appears to a police officer that use of firearms may be imminent. The general rule taught at police academies is: when you draw your weapon, place your index finger along the frame of your firearm and keep it there. You don't let your finger enter the trigger guard or rest on the trigger until you decide to shoot.[262] If the finger stays outside the trigger guard, there is no worry about accidentally or involuntarily discharging the weapon by pulling the trigger. Every officer knows and understands the rule, yet unintended discharges continue to happen. The problem, after considerable research by Page and his associates, is that even experienced officers put their finger on the trigger before they have made the decision to shoot, without any awareness that they are doing so.[263]

In one training session, Page utilized a shooting video with a standard circle drawing as the target, with a chime signal for an officer to draw, and a buzzer signaling when to shoot. The defined purpose was announced for the shooter to not put his finger on the trigger until the buzzer sounded. The captain and ten trained officers all failed the test, despite constant reminders to "Keep your finger off the trigger until the buzzer sounds." Fingers on the trigger are a recipe for unintended actions. This literal statement works as an apt metaphor for the rest of us when communicating: Keep your finger off the trigger until time to "fire."

Self-Talk provided a cure for officer premature shootings. The captain and other officers were taught to say the word "finger" out loud when the weapon was drawn and repeated until the buzzer sounded. All officers succeeded in keeping their fingers out of the trigger guard on every trial using this technique. Extensive subsequent practice was needed to make the thinking and the response automatic.[264]

Mental Imagery as a Tool for Cognitive Control

Mental imagery is important for developing your plan of action for behaviors you wish to change. By mentally visualizing your plan of action, you can anticipate the kind of action you want to develop. Athletes picture themselves being successful, noting all the details that need to be addressed.[265] Behavioral problems can likewise be addressed and corrected through visualization and self-talk. "Raymond," for example, had the habit of reaching for and devouring a large bag of potato chips when he felt hungry after dinner. He pictured himself reaching instead for fruit, such as grapes or an apple. He devised the code-word "salt" when he was tempted, took a deep breath, and over time became satisfied with the healthier substitute. In Chapter 12, we introduced Sam, who had a similar problem. What advice would you now give Sam?

Cognitive control involves setting and reaching goals. In order to be successful in school and in life, you must complete tasks at hand such as solving a difficult problem despite the temptation to give up and watch TV instead. This kind of cognitive control is necessary to deal with such problems as addiction, bad habits, and harmful impulses. Often to succeed in life you must work toward a long-term goal at the expense of short-term ones. For example, choosing to go to graduate school may involve the delayed gratification of a good salary for an even better one when graduate school is completed. This kind of control has been demonstrated to produce such results as better grades, higher credit ratings, better mental and emotional health, and better interpersonal functioning, which results in better relationships, stronger family cohesion, and better skills in handling emotional issues (such as anger).

You can use cognitive control in response to situations that have in the past caused you to resort to defensive responses. You can replace them with appropriate and healthier supportive responses. Planning and intention must be formulated.

Mindfulness Meditation

Mindfulness meditation is an exercise in attention. An all-around healthy practice, it is especially effective in retraining automatic responses that are defensive, unhelpful, or self-defeating. It involves calming the mind, typically by focusing on the breath, as in the Jonathan Page program. Begin by identifying the situation or "trigger" for a specific unhealthy response. Set aside a period of time in which you can be free of stress and that situation. Now imagine the stressor or trigger. Use this time to observe all the things in your field of awareness with unusual care and clarity. In the calm of the moment, listen for sounds, note the colors in your surroundings and what you are feeling. Since feelings have such a profound effect on our perceptions, thoughts, and behavior, treat them skeptically. Reflect on them and decide which ones to trust. Do your emotions filter your perceptions, distorting your view of reality? Take a moment before taking any action or reaching a judgment.

You may be anxious about a scheduled future event. You may dread a social gathering with people you don't know very well. Picture someone you would like to know better who will be there. Meditation, as described in ancient texts, makes people more aware of their feelings and less likely to be reflexively governed by them. As Robert Wright says, "This remains a central goal of mindfulness meditation today."[266]

Go back over the reflections and activities that you felt were meaningful. Do you have a sense of accomplishment? Think about changes you have made or still want to make.

Unlocking Your Future with Healthy Communication

Tips for Greater Authenticity. Authenticity is inherently tied to reality, truth, and trust. An old Buddhist parable describes a wise man teaching his grandson. The wise man tells him that there are two wolves battling inside every person. One is filled with arrogance, greed, anger, manipulation, and hatred, the other with honesty, peace, generosity, humility, and goodwill. "Which wolf will win?" asks the grandson. The wise man replies, "The one you feed."[267]

The desire for authenticity in your life is a lifelong quest. When you are authentic, you not only acknowledge the truth of your feelings, needs and wishes, but you are capable of congruency in your close personal relationships. You can enter into true dialogue spontaneously without defenses or reserve. This experience of revealing your true self to another permits you to know yourself better.

The best advice we offer is to experiment with authentic self-disclosure cautiously with tact and a loving, trusting heart. Authentic being and authentic self-disclosure are necessary factors in the attainment of healthy communication.

Tips for Greater Empathy. We have emphasized how important it is for young children to learn empathic skills. Adults also may wish to hone their empathy skills.

You can sharpen your listening skills. You may need to not offer advice, only to listen and share a significant other's mood, feelings, and concerns with patience and shared emotions. Focus on the similarities you share. Don't interrupt or change the subject. At the end of a difficult day, your spouse may just need time to vent. He/she may just want you to understand and share their feelings, rather than want you to "fix it."

You must be able to listen with acceptance and validation. When you truly listen and offer supportive responses, the partner will be able to open up even more. Empathy should lead to understanding and reduced stress. A former student of one of the authors had this to say about the transforming consequences of being listened to and truly heard.

> A number of times in my life, I have felt confronted by seemingly unsolvable problems, overcome by feelings of worthlessness and despair. I've been fortune to have been with people who have

been available to me and even been able to hear my meanings more deeply than I did myself. They just listened, clarified and responded to me without passing judgement on me, without taking responsibility or offering excuses and without trying to mold me. It felt damn good. It relaxed the tension in me, permitting me to bring out the feelings, the guilt, the fears and the confusion that had been past experience. When I was listened to, truly heard, I was able to re-perceive my world, the unsolvable became solvable and confusions became clear. I have appreciated deeply the time that I have experienced this sensitive, empathic concerted listening.

As an exercise, empathize with someone who is volunteering and helping others. Ask what rewards they are getting out of the experience. State your honest appreciation for their service. In a similar exercise, when you are feeling happy and in a wonderful mood, share it with others. Notice the reciprocity in a smile and shared happiness. Notice how sharing happiness often increases the enjoyment.

Tips for Empowerment. Empowerment is the true vehicle for growth, whether for an individual, a relationship, or an organization. Some business leaders know that when they give employees the opportunity to utilize their creative, analytical, and problem-solving abilities, they are more productive due to the level of trust placed in them. Shared purpose and a greater feeling of importance with team work are typical results of personal empowerment.

Check yourself when you are tempted to complain. If you are a leader, look for opportunities to delegate and to create decision-making tasks at lower levels. If you are not in a position of leadership and are feeling an absence of power, identify the power that you do have. Seek ways to make necessary changes. Talk to the right person or institute a change for yourself. Complaints to the wrong parties simply stir up discontent. Many professional organizations now offer workshops and educational programs designed to promote empowerment.

We have cited research that shows community empowerment leads to improved health and well-being. Empowerment strategies are more likely to be successful if they are incorporated within wider macro-economic and policy strategies aimed at promoting greater equality. Coordination with existing community organizations and agencies is needed to gain maximum support. Funding, support mechanisms, and development opportunities should be in place. Both the professional community and the people being served must "be on the same page."

This movement toward greater empowerment of groups seeking change has spread internationally. Here are three examples:

1. A child-nutrition program in Vietnam empowered women to share information and learn problem-solving and childcare skills in

supportive environments, leading to better food intake for the children, more immunizations, reduced depression related to illnesses, and a reduction in such unhealthy behaviors as overeating and drug and alcohol abuse.[268]

2. Participative learning exercises in women's groups in rural Nepal resulted in a reduction in neonatal and maternal mortality. Through the group participation, the women became able to define, analyze, and then, through the support of others, articulate and promote their support needs regarding childbirth to policy makers.[269]

3. Empowerment strategies aimed at such high-risk groups as sex workers and injecting drug users resulted in behavioral changes.[270] Similarly, evidence produced from evaluations of youth empowerment interventions revealed increased participation in social actions and actual policy changes linked to improved health and educational outcomes.[271]

Practicing Healthy Communication

1. Meet with your closest friend and tell her/him of your plan: to devote a couple of hours to honestly exploring in depth your true feelings and future goals. Focus on being fully honest, attempting to fully understand each other's feelings as well as ideas. Listen carefully and seek total clarity. Exhibit your full, unconditional regard for the other.

2. Make an effort to talk to someone with whom you have only an impersonal relationship. You may have been around this neighbor, co-worker, or service provider for some time and never gotten to know him/her – sometimes not even his/her name. Engage them for a moment of genuinely healthy communication. Express your appreciation for their presence in your life and demonstrate interest in them and their lives. You both will be richer for the moment.

3. Mend a fence with someone with whom you feel alienated. Initiate contact with this person and tell them that you miss them and wish to reconnect. *Practice healthy communication!*

4. Conduct an assessment of your personal needs for success, feelings of contentment, pleasure and happiness. Talk to a trusted other and form a plan of action to address your own needs.

5. Identify habits you want to change, emotional triggers that result in unwanted results, and unhealthy behaviors that need to be addressed. Create a plan of action.

6. Have your hearing tested. Hearing loss has been labeled "America's silent epidemic." The young as well as the older are afflicted. Hearing loss is associated with an increased risk of depression, social isolation,

loneliness, falls and dementia. Nearly 30% of people in their fifties, 45% in their sixties and 65% in their seventies have significant hearing loss that too often is undiagnosed.

7. Conduct a healthy communication audit of your interactions with others. Are you in unhealthy relationships? What actions will contribute to your greater health and the greater health of all your relationships?

8. Remember that you don't want to control communication with partners, family and friends but you want to interact in supportive ways, controlling your words and deeds so others may interact with you honestly and openly.

9. Try a new hobby or leisure activity. If your lifestyle is sedentary, try an exercise class or a sport. Consider some leisure activity that is diametrically opposed to your vocation. If you lead a busy, socially engaged professional life, a solitary leisure pastime such as reading, painting or playing a musical instrument can be invaluable. If you have solitary work, be with others in your after-work activities.

10. Consider your use of the word "can't" when you discover yourself saying "I can't" (for example, "I can't break up with him" or "I can't make her understand.") There's a good chance you are making a choice ("I choose not to break up with him.") It may be a simple matter of not knowing how to proceed ("I don't know how to make her understand.") Recognizing the difference between choices, missing knowledge and real limitations (in reality, I can't lift a two-ton car) empowers you with a potential course of action (I can still tow that two-ton car).

11. Exercise your power to influence local, state and national politics by staying aware of current issues and voting.

12. Be involved in improving the world around you by volunteering.

13. Empower yourself by separating facts from unsupported assertions, interpretations, and perspectives in your personal, interpersonal and social lives. Don't confuse your interpretations of another's behavior with their actual behavior. Separate factual information from viral stories spread throughout the internet. Hold news sources accountable for sharing accurate information. When in doubt, check sources before jumping to accept, respond, or reach conclusions.

In review, personal, relational and societal health consists of action rather than a state. You are physically healthy when you can process food, water and air to expend energy doing what you wish. You are emotionally healthy when you are capable of solving personal problems and living a rich life. Your relationships are healthy when you are open and empathic with others. Similarly, healthy societies exist when individuals unite to guarantee satisfaction of physical, emotional and safety needs of members by sharing resources and resolving conflicts in a peaceful process that engenders trust and good will. Healthy societies protect their membership through peaceful interactions with other societies. Be Healthy!

Appendix A: Fact Checks—Useful Resources on the Internet

The Duke Reporters Lab reports that there are now 341 fact checkers in the world that produce organized fact-checking in a journalistic fashion. Over half of those fact checkers are affiliated with media organizations. Others are associated with not-for-profit groups, NGO's, think-tanks or academic institutions. Some have multiple affiliations. Fact checkers exist in at least 102 countries and issue reports in nearly 70 languages.

All fact checkers are not equal though; some may have hidden agendas, lazy research practices, biased topic selection or reporting, or resort to lying in their checks simply to cast doubt on truthful people. Some are responsible to those who pay their paychecks or a suppressive government in which they must survive. Trustworthy fact checkers openly state their objectives and provide the sources of their reports so you can check original facts yourself. It is logical that those who point out the dishonesty of others will find themselves embroiled in controversy occasionally. You'll have to decide who presents truths based on facts, who displays bias by only investigating facts they oppose, the resources they cite, their logic, and their reputation. Those were the considerations used to determine the following resources.

The International Fact Checking Network (IFCN) sets a code of principles that must be followed in order to remain a part of the network. Those requirements include non-partisanship, impartiality, transparency, listing resources, and methodology of checking as well as listing how they are funded on their website. IFCN signatories are indicated on the following list. You can see applications and a list of members on the IFCN web site. Those sites that are not IFCN signatories have been included as they have established their credibility in other ways.

AFP Fact Check (IFCN) <https://factcheck.afp.com>
The Agence France-Presse (AFP) is an international news agency based in France with locations around the globe. International fact checks are available for countries other than the USA.

Funding: About 2/3 of AFP funding comes from commercial backing. Other funds are provided from a French government subsidy to support impartial, public interest journalism in France and abroad.

Subjects covered: diverse subjects, photos and videos from many countries.

All Sides (IFCN) <AllSides.com>
This site dedicates itself to exposing bias and providing multiple perspectives on issues. Labels stories as left leaning, center, or right leaning. A good resource for seeing how different political sides "spin" the same facts.

Funding: Uses a for profit business model. Donors include liberals (Tom Steyer) and conservatives (Charles Koch).

Subjects covered: Politics.

AltNews (IFCN) <http://altnews.in>

This is one of the few fact-checking websites in India which is certified by the IFC. Fights fake news in India by revealing fake claims and political misinformation with technological help and on-ground reports. Offers information in both English and Hindi. Partners with WhatsApp to bust fake news on its chat platform and debunks claims made on social media platforms.

Funding: Run by Pravda Media Foundation, but funding is primarily user donations and independent media trusts.

Subjects covered: Debunks claims made on social media platforms covering science, education and society at large._

AP Fact Check (IFCN) Http://apnews.com/hub/fact-checking

Associated Press's website is an independent global news organization dedicated to factual reporting. Founded in 1846, it is trusted to provide news and sources to many trustworthy newspapers.

Funding: Independent global news organization.

Subjects covered: political leaders' statements.

Boom FactCheck <https://www.boomlive.in>

This fact checking site, located in India, exposes fake news on digital platforms. It is run by Data journalist, Govindraf Ethiraj, who worked for Bloomberg prior to coming to FactCheck, and offers service in English, Hindi, and Bengali.

Funding: Ads and user donations. Boom is part of Ping Digital Network, a private limited company head quartered in Mumbai, India. The website is funded by Ping and its investors.

Subjects covered: Covers current news cycle, political rhetoric, claims running viral on social media, urban legends, myths, and rumors.

Check Your Fact (IFCN) https://checkyourfact.com

This is one of the few right-leaning IFCN fact checkers.

Funding: Owned by the Daily Caller, but working independently of them.

Subjects covered: Hoaxes and Political Statements.

FactCheck.Org (IFCN) < http://www.factcheck.org/> #FactCheckorg

This non-partisan/non-profit site attempts to bring accountability to public officials by exposing deception and lies. They say their purposes are to "apply the best practices of both journalism and scholarship and to increase public knowledge and understanding." They annually print that year's most egregious claims in their "Whoppers of the Year." The site confirms the reliability of sources consulted and shares that information with readers.

Funding: Run by the Annenberg Public Policy Center of the University of Pennsylvania and primarily funded by the Annenberg Foundation, a nonprofit organization.

Subjects covered: Political claims and rhetoric made by the president, members of congress, presidential candidates and other members of the political arena. Statements might be made in TV ads, speeches, debates, interviews, and news releases.

Fact-Checker Bot by IFCN (Poynter Institute's International Fact-Checkers Network) on WhatsApp

Fact Checker Bot lets you check facts and get connected with fact-checkers in your region so you can check local news. They offer latest fact-check message alerts that can save you time and needless aggravation by reaching you prior to unsubstantiated or just plain fabricated stories.

To use: Send a "Hi" message to +1(727)2912606.

Fact Tank: News in the Numbers (found on the Pew research website) <http://pewresearch.org/>

This is run by the Pew Research Center which describes itself as "a nonpartisan fact tank that informs the public about the issues, attitudes and trends shaping the world.

Funding: Pew Research Center.

Subjects covered: The research center conducts and reports public opinion polls, demographic research, media content analysis and other empirical social science research.

Full Fact (IFCN) <https.fullfact.org>

Full Fact is based in the UK and is especially helpful checking information in Europe. A team of independent fact-checkers and volunteers find viral posts from social media and expose them to keep them from misleading people using the internet. Full Fact runs a "Viral Posts on Facebook" page listing outrageous claims and debunks them with detailed explanation and authentic sources. The UK's version of the US's Politifact.

Funding: Independent/nonprofit.

Subjects covered: Wide variety of subjects with focus on political claims and misinformation published by the UK media: provides well researched and resourced articles. Resources include academic and professional papers.

Lead Stories (IFCN) <https://leadstories.com>

This award-winning site uses a specific engine called the Trendolizer tracking stories and trends that allow the site to debunk fake news before it becomes viral.

Funding: funded in part by Chinese company ByteDance LLC, (owner of TikTok) and has been accused of censorship on behalf of the country's communist government.

Subjects covered: Hoaxes, outrageous claims, and rumors.

Media Bias/Fact Check (IFCN) <http:// mediabiasfactcheck.com>

This is a comprehensive media bias resource.

Funding: Advertising (60 percent) memberships of $2, $5, or $10 per month (36 percent). Donations from individuals only (4 percent), A collective of volunteers and paid contractors help keep the costs low.

Subjects covered: More than 3200 media sources are listed in their database. More are added daily.

Media Matters for America < https://mediamatters.org>>

This liberal web-based, non-profit research and information center is dedicated to comprehensively monitoring analyzing and correcting misinformation in the U.S. media."

Funding: Individual donors, George Soros personally and through his partnerships with other groups and federally backed small business loans as part of the Paycheck Protection Program during the 2020 COVID-19 pandemic.

Subjects covered: Conservative Media Reports (especially FOX news since 2011) but also checks broadcast, radio, print for factual errors.

News Busters < https://www.newsbusters.org>

This site combats liberal media bias. It has been criticized for its questionable fact-checking techniques.

Funding: Launched in 2005 by the Media Research Center (the same group behind CNS News.com.), it receives financial support from several right-leaning sources including the Bradley, Scaife, Olin, Castle Rock, Carthage, J Foundations and Exxon Mobil. Funded by MRC and displays advertising.

Subjects covered: liberal news reports.

OpenSecrets <https://www.opensecrets.org/> #OpenSecrets

This site identifies the effects of money lobbying in politics by tracking how a politician is funded and which firms are funneling money into politics. Since it was begun in 1983, it is one of the largest public databases of donors and political beneficiaries.

Funding: Run by the Center for Responsive Politics which is both non-profit and non-partisan.

Subjects covered: Traces the money trail in politics, lists where politicians get their money, reports on PACs and exposes the underbelly of dark money, useful in understanding the effect of lobbying in US politics.

PolitiFact (IFCN) <http://politifact,com/ #PolitiFact

This is one of the largest political fact-checking newsrooms in the US and received a 2008 Pulitzer Prize for National Reporting. They rate statements with a spectrum of choices ranging from True, Mostly True, Half True, False and "Pants on Fire."

Funding: run by the Poynter Institute (founder of International Fact-Checking Network) and reporters from the Independent Tampa Bay Times.

Subjects checked: Claims that might be heard in politician's speeches or television ads or on-line political party rants.

ProPublica_<htpps://www.propublica.org>

This is an independent online newsroom known for its investigative journalism. It has created one of the largest local reporting networks which means information from all parts of the country breaks accurately and quickly. The web site has received many prestigious awards including six Pulitzer Prizes for public service, explanatory reporting, national reporting, and investigative journalism.

Funding: The Knight Foundation, MacArthur Foundation, Ford Foundation, and other philanthropic institutes.

Subjects covered: Covers practically any subject that is of public interest: politics, healthcare, education, finances, criminal justice.

PunditFact (IFCN) <www.politifact.com/punditfact/>

As a project of the Poynter Institute, PunditFact is dedicated to checking the accuracy of claims by pundits, columnists, bloggers, political analysts, the hosts and guests of talk shows, and other members of the media.

Funding: PunditFact is funded in part by $625,000 in grants over two years from the Ford Foundation and the Democracy Fund and ads.

Subjects covered: Assertions made by individuals as a matter of public mediated mass record.

Reuters Fact Check *(IFCN)* < https://reuters.com/factcheck

This is a UK based fact checker that provides sources.

Funding: Thomson Reuters Foundation and others including academic, foundations, non-profits, industry partners, and earned income from leadership development programs and other activities.

Subjects covered: social media hoaxes and claims, as well as political statements.

SciCheck <https://factcheck.org/scicheck/>
Fact Check's site was launched in 2015 and focuses exclusively on false and misleading scientific claims that are made by politicians to influence public policy.

Funding: their COVID-19 *Misconception's* page is made possible by a Robert Wood Johnson Foundation—subscribers and donors. SciCheck publicly discloses anyone who makes a donation of $1000 or more by posting quarterly financial statements available on their website and e-mails them to subscribers.

Subjects covered: Scientific claims used by politicians of any party as support for arguments constructed to influence public policy.

Science Feedback (IFCN) <https://sciencefeedback.co>
This has two separate websites, Climate Feedback and Health Feedback. Fact checkers are scientists holding Ph.Ds. who have recently published in top tier peer reviewed scientific journals.

Subjects covered: climate related claims are directed to Climate Feedback and health and medical claims are directed to Health Feedback.

SM Hoax Slayer <https://www.smhoaxslayer.com>
This web site seeks to expose fake information on social media platforms by debunking claims and updating users through its social media channels. The project started by investigating harmless lies, pranks, and rumors, but soon developed into a fact checking website. Many mainstream newspapers and media houses cite SM Hoax Slayer as a reliable source.

Funding: Mostly run by volunteers and funded by user donations and ads.

Subjects covered: debunks memes, fake videos, and internet hoaxes, especially those shared on Facebook.

Snopes <https://www.Snopes.com>
This is one of the oldest authoritative fact-checking websites on the internet. Checks offer detailed explanations from reliable sources such as the World Health Organization or the National Center for Disease Control and experts holding impressive credentials and recognized by others in their respective fields.

Funding: Relying on grants, ads, and donations for funding.

Subjects covered: site deals with practically everything (politics, history, science, health, and technology) and offers checks for urban myths, stories, rumors, hoaxes, half-truths and outrageous claims.

Sunlight Foundation <https://sunlightfoundation.com>

This web site is a national, nonpartisan, nonprofit organization that uses civic technologies, open data, policy analysis and journalism to make our government and politics more accountable and transparent to all.

Funding: Ownership funds. The Sunlight Foundation is a 501(c)(3), nonprofit that accepts donations from liberal and conservative sources. Before accepting donations over $250, the offer is scrutinized to ensure that the donations will not influence fact checking results. Donors include the Open Society Foundations, The Pew Charitable Trusts, the John S. and James L. Knight Foundation, the Rockefeller Foundation, the Ford Foundation, the William and Flora Hewlett Foundation, the Omidyar Network, Bloomberg Philanthropies, and the Laura and John Arnold Foundation. The website openly discloses their largest donors.

Subjects covered: government actions and politics.

Tin Eye < https://tineye.com>

This web site provides a reverse image search which tells whether or not an image was altered.

Funding: Clients pay—Independent, self-funded.

Subjects covered: Photos and images.

Washington Post Fact Checker (IFCN) <https://www.washingtonpost.com/news/fact-checker/>

This web site presents critical analysis of what politicians have said in a current week. Left bias is shown as they investigate more right-wing claims than left, however, their fact checks are excellent and sourced.

Funding: one of the few fact-checking columns run by a mainstream media house.

Subjects covered: Facts and contexts against seemingly truthful narratives presented in politics or viral stories. Especially useful in determining "fake news." Fake news is not just about something that is not true; sometimes it establishes narratives that are counter to the sum of the facts.

Appendix B: Trustworthy News Sources

It is important to note that in 2020 five companies controlled 90 percent of the United States media. Each of the following has been listed by at least two evaluators for presenting unbiased accurate news stories. They meet journalistic requirements of fair factual reporting, and when they are judged to lean either to the left or the right, it is because of subject choice rather than a bias in writing. This is not an exhaustive list. You will be able to vet sources for yourself.

ASSOCIATED PRESS has garnered 53 Pulitzer Prizes.

BBC is the world's oldest and one of the largest national broadcasting services in the world.

THE BUREAU OF INVESTIGATIVE JOURNALISM (for British politics).

THE CHRISTIAN SCIENCE MONITOR

C-SPAN allows you to watch government hearings and events directly.

THE ECONOMIST

FAIR is a watchdog group that writes about media bias, and is noted for fairness and accuracy in reporting.

THE FINANCIAL TIMES

NATIONAL PUBLIC RADIO—A Pew survey shows that conservatives tend to mistrust NPR, but its journalistic values are high and it is known for rejecting sensationalism, fair reporting and issuing corrections as problems are noted.

PEW RESEARCH is a non-partisan think tank that publishes pure facts and figures frequently used in news reports.

PROPUBLICA is the first online news organization to win a Pulitzer Prize. Others have followed.

REUTERS—AllSides, Media Bias Fact Check and *The Economist* reports all rate Reuters to be one of the most unbiased news sources available.

USA TODAY

THE WALL STREET JOURNAL AllSides confirms unbiased news coverage with a slight lean to the right-center. A 2014 Pew Research Center Study found that the *Wall Street Journal* tends to provide equal coverage across the political spectrum.

NEW YORK TIMES along with the *Wall Street Journal* and *USA TODAY* have the highest readership.

ABC, CBS, and **NBC** are network news stations that do not have as many mentions for accuracy and unbiased reporting as those listed above, but are never-the-less considered trustworthy sources.

Endnotes

Chapter 1

[1] Chris Segrin, *Interpersonal Processes in Psychological Problems* (New York: Guilford, 2001) vii.

[2] Nidal Moukanddam and Asim Sham, "Psychologists Beware! The Impact of COVID-19 and Pandemics on Mental Health," *Psychiatric Times*, 37, 4 (March 15, 2020) 1-7. *The New York Times*, April 9, 2020.

[3] www.cdc.gov/violenceprevention/acestudy

[4] Daniel Goleman, *Emotional Intelligence: Why It Can Matter More than Intelligence* (New York: Bantam Dell, 2006) 4-10.

[5] Rebecca Banks, "Health and the Spiritual Dimension," *Journal of School Health* 50, 4 (1980): 198, 195-202.

[6] John Pilch, "Wellness Spirituality," *Health Values* 12 (1988): 28-31.

[7] Larry Chapman, "Developing a Useful Perspective on Spiritual Health," *American Journal of Health Promotion* 1 (1987): 12-17.

[8] Banks, Ibid.

[9] S. Hawk, "Spiritual Health: Definition and Theory," *Wellness Perspectives* 10, 4 (1994): 3-14.

[10] Abraham Maslow, *Motivation and Personality* (New York: Harper & Row, 1970).

[11] Larry Chapman, "Health: A Component Missing from Health Promotion," *American Journal of Health Promotion* 1 (1986): 38-41.

[12] Carol D. Ryff and Berton H. Singer, eds., *Emotion, Social Relationships, and Health* (New York: Oxford University Press, 2001) 3.

[13] Bert N. Uchino, *Social Support and Physical Health* (New Haven: Yale University Press, 2004) 17.

[14] Richard E. Lucas and P. S. Dyrenforth, "Does the Existence of Social Relationships Matter for Subjective Well-Being?" in *Self and Relationship*, eds, Kathleen D. Vohs and Eli J. Finkel (New York: Guilford Press, 2006) 254-258.

[15] Michael Argyle, *The Psychology of Happiness* (New York: Methuen, 2006) 223.

[16] *Journal of Clinical Psychiatry*, January 2016, cited in *USA Today*, January 27, 2016.

[17] Brett Molina, "Health Insurer: More Americans Depressed," *USA Today*, May 14, 2018, 18.

[18] Ibid.

[19] Teresa Seeman, "How Do Others Get Under Our Skin?" *Emotion, Social Relationships and Health* (New York: Oxford University Press, 2001) 204.

[20] Steven A. Schroeder, "We Can Do Better in Improving the Health of the American People," *The New England Journal of Medicine*, September 20, 2007, 1221-1228.

[21] Ibid., 1222.

Chapter 2

[22] Jurgen Ruesch, *Therapeutic Communication* (New York: Norton, 1961).

[23] Bert N. Uchino, *Social Support and Physical Health* (New Haven: Yale University Press, 2004).

[24] Rollo May, *Man's Search for Himself* (New York: Norton, 1953) 75.

[25] Mirsa, Shalini., Cheng, Lulu, Genevie, Jamie, and Yuan, Miao. (2014). "The iPhone effect: The quality of in-person social interactions in the presence of mobile devices." *Environment & Behavior*; Andrew K. Przybylski, Netta Weinstein. (2013). "Can you connect with me now? How the presence of mobile communication technology influences face-to-face conversational quality". *Journal of Social and Personal Relationships*, 30, 237-246.

[26] Miriam Horston, Martin Middleman, and S.P. Wamala "Psychosocial Factors and Heart Rate Variability in Healthy Women," *Psychosomatic Medicine* 61 (1999): 49-57.

[27] Uchino, 58.

[28] Ibid., 88.

[29] Ibid., 89-93.

[30] Ibid., 94-97.

[31] Ibid., 97

[32] Sheldon Cohen, "Social Relationships and Susceptibility to the Common Cold" in *Emotions, Social Relationships and Health*, 122-126.

[33] Ibid.

[34] Ibid., 221-242.

[35] Sheldon Cohen, "Happy People are Healthier," Nov. 2006 at www.psychosomaticmedicine.org.

[36] Uchino, 182.

Chapter 3

[37]Michio Kaku, *The Future of the Mind* (New York: Doubleday, 2014) 20.

[38]Alek Korb, *The Upward Spiral* (CA: New Harbinger Publications, Inc., 2015) 3-4.

[39]Ibid., 13-14

[40]Louis Cozolino, *The Neuroscience of Human Relationships* (New York: W. W. Norton and Company, 2013).

[41]Ibid., 225-260.

[42]Jenna Gallegos, "The Development of Your Child's Brain," *Washington Post*, reprinted in *Kansas City Star*, September 3, 2017, 20A.

[43]Ibid.

[44]Ibid.

[45]Ibid.

[46]Roy F. Baumeister, "Self-Control Requires Energy That Needs to be Restored," *Alcoholism: Clinical and Experimental Research* 27, 2, (2003): 15

[47]Liane Leedom, *Just Like His Father? A Guide to Overcoming Your Child's Genetic Connection to Antisocial Behavior, Addiction and ADHD (*Fairfield, CT: Healing Arts Press LLC, 2006).

[48]J. David Hawkins, Ray Catalano, and Gerald Miller, "Early Effects of Communities That Care on Targeted Risks and Initiation of Delinquent Behavior and Substance Use," *Journal of Adolescent Health*, 43, 1 (2008): 15-22.

[49]Baumeister.

[50]Ibid.

[51]Gardner's ideas as explained by Karl Albrecht, *Social Intelligence: The New Science of Success* (San Francisco: Jossey-Bass, 2006) xii-xiii.

[52]Ibid.

[53]Daniel Goleman, *Emotional Intelligence* (New York: Bantam Dell, 1994).

[54]Ibid.

Chapter 4

[55]Francis Crick, cited by Steven Pinker, "The Mystery of Consciousness," *Time*. 169, 5 (January 29, 2007) 59-62.

[56]R. D. Laing, *The Politics of Experience* (New York: Ballantine, 1967).

[57]Bobby R. Patton and Kim Giffin, *Interpersonal Communication in Action* (New York: Harper & Row, 1977) 165-167.

[58]Timothy Snyder, *The Road to Unfreedom* (New York: Tom Duggan Books, 2018) 11.

[59]Ibid., 246.

[60]Steven Pinker, The Stuff of Thought (New York: Viking, 2007) 435.

[61] Hans Rosling, *Factfulness* (New York: Flatiron Books, 2018).

[62]Carl R. Rogers, "What It Means to Become a Person." In C. E. Moustakas, ed., *The Self* (New York: Harper & Row, 1959) 197.

[63]Carl R. Rogers. *On Becoming a Person* (Boston: Houghton Mifflin, 1961) 338-346.

[64]Sidney Jourard. *The Transparent Self* (New York: Van Nostrand Reinhold, 1964) 184-185.

[65]Ervine Goffman. "On Face-Work: An Analysis of Ritual Elements in Social Interaction," *Psychiatry*, 18 (1955): 213-231.

[66]Ervine Goffman. *The Presentation of Self in Everyday Life* (Garden City, N.Y.: Doubleday, 1959).

[67]Ibid., 6-14.

[68]Paul Watzlawick, Janet Beavin and Don D. Jackson, *Pragmatics of Communication* (New York: Norton, 1967) 62-67.

[69]Sidney M. Jourard, *Healthy Personality* (New York: Macmillan Publishing Co., 1963) 156-162.

[70]Ibid., 157.

[71]Ibid., 159.

Chapter 5

[72] Ibid.

[73] Amy Biolchini, "How Talking Politics with Oprah Winfrey Changed Grand Rapids-Area Voters." (https://www.mlive.com/news/grandrapids/2017/09/how_talking_politics_with_opra.html), September. 25, 2017 Updated: May, 20 2019

[74] Ibid.

[75] Ibid.

186

[76] 60 Minutes: Oprah follows up with the partisan voters in Michigan about Donald Trump - CBS News. February. 18, 2018. Produced by Tanya Simon, Graham Messick, Magalie Laguerre-Wilkinson and Jack Weingart. CBS Interactive Inc.

[77] Wikipedia, https://en.wikipedia.org.

[78] Joseph Uscinski, "Clean Thinking About Conspiracy Theories in Troubled Times," *Skeptical Inquirer*, 45, No. 1, January/February, 2021, 52-56.

[79] Ibid.

[80] Ibid.

[81] Russel Falcon, NEXSTAR Media Wire, posted November 3, 2021, reported on Fox News (KXAN).

[82] William C. Schutz, *The Interpersonal Underworld* (Palo Alto, CA: Science and Behavior Books, 1966) 13-33

[83] Eric Berne, *Games People Play* (New York: Grove Press, 1964).

[84] Sidney M. Jourard, *Healthy Personality* (New York: Macmillan, 1974) 239.

[85] Subia Rasheed, "Self-Awareness as a Therapeutic Tool," *International Journal of Caring Sciences*, January-April 2015, 211-215.

[86] Kathleen Verderber and Rudolph Verderber, *Interpersonal Communication Concepts, Skills and Contexts*, (New York: Oxford University Press – 10th edition, 2004) pp 245-247.

[87] Sharon S. Brehm, *Intimate Relationships* (New York: Random House, 1985) 216-217.

[88] Jourard, 225.

[89] William B. Gudykunst and Young Yun Kim, *Communicating with Strangers: An Approach to Intercultural Communication* (Boston; Allyn and Bacon, 2007).

[90] Kristen Fuller, "Intimate Violence and Child Abuse During COVID-19," *Psychology* on line, 16 April 2020.

[91] Joselyn Noveck, "With Isolation, Domestic Abuse Activists Fear 'Explosive Cocktail,' Associated Press, 26 April 2020.

[92] Sid Kirchheimer, *AARP Bulletin*, July - August 2007, 26.

[93] Zlati Meyer, *USA Today*, 9 March 2017.

[94] Villarreal Alexandra. *Guardian*, 26 May 2021.

[95] "2015 Stress in America Survey." American Psychological Association. www.apa.org.

[96] Jaime M. Grant, Lisa Mottet and Justin Tanis, National Center for Transgender Equality and the National Gay and Lesbian Task Force, October, 2010.

[97] I.Meyer, "Prejudice, Social Stress, and Mental Health in Lesbian, Gay, and Bisexual Populations: Conceptual Issues and Research Evidence." *Psychological Bulletin* 129 (2003): 674-697.

[98] Benjamin Radford, "Coronavirus Crisis: Confronting Our Biases," *Skeptical Inquiry*, 44, No. 4, April 23, 2020.

[99] Colleen Long, Michael Balsamo, and Rodney Muhumuza, "Coronavirus-related Crimes Capitalize on Global Fear and the Urge to Blame," *Time*, April 11, 2020

[100] Ibid.

[101] Ibid.

[102] Ibid.

[103] Belinda Luscombe, "Retired General Stanley McChrystal Believe Our Leaders can do Better," *Time*, October 25/November 1, 2021, 20.

[104] Roger Shepard, *Mind Sights: Original Visual Illusions, Ambiguities, and Other Anomalies, With a Commentary of the Play of Mind in Perception and Art* (New York: Freeman, 1990).

[105] Tim Rizzo, "Convicted Man Freed after Search turns up his Doppelganger," *Kansas City Star*, 10 June 2017, 4 A.

[106] Doug Chayka, "He Predicted the 2016 Fake News Crisis. Now he's Worried about an Information Apocalypse," *Buzz Feed News*, 11 February 2018.

[107] Kim Giffin and Richard Barnes, *Trusting Me, Trusting You* (Columbus, OH: Charles E. Merrill Publishing Co., 1976) 7.

[108] Stephen M. R. Covey, *The Speed of Trust, The One Thing That Changes Everything* (New York: The Free Press, 2006).

[109] Don Peppers and Martha Rogers, *Extreme Trust: Honesty as a Competitive Advantage* (New York: Portfolio/Penguin, 2012).

[110] Ibid.

[111] Greg Gigerenzer, *Risk Savvy – How to Make Good Decisions* (New York: Viking, 2014).

[112] Ibid., 261.

[113] Steve Hartman, "Girl Scout Takes on the Mantle of Truth in Advertising," CBS Evening News, February 17, 2017.

Chapter 7

[114]Associated Press, Monday, January 21, 2008.

[115]Elizabeth Segal, M. Alex Wagaman and Karen Gerdes, "Developing the Social Empathy Index: An Exploratory Factor Analysis," *Advances in Social Work.* 13, 3, 2012.

[116]Emma Seppala "Connect to Thrive: Social Connection Improves Health, Well-Being & Longevity." *Psychology Today*, https:/www.psychologytoday.com/blog/feeling-it/201208/connect-thrive.

[117]Ervin Staub "Commentary on Part I [Historical and Theoretical Perspectives] in *Empathy and Its Development*, eds. Nancy Eisenberg and Jane Strayer (New York: Cambridge University Press, 1987) 109-113.

[118]Ross Buck and Benson Ginsburg, "Communicative Genes and the Evolution of Empathy," in *Empathic Accuracy*, ed. Willian Ickes (New York: The Guilford Press, 1997) 17-43.

[119]Robert Plutchik, "Evolutionary Bases of Empathy," in *Empathy and Its Development*, eds. Nancy Eisenberg and Jane Strayer (New York: Cambridge University Press, 1987) 45.

[120]Marshall Rosenberg, "Benefits" as cited by Center for Building a Culture of Empathy, retrieved from http://cultureofempathy.com/References/Benefits/Articles.htm

[121]Samuel Natale, *An Experiment in Empathy* (Great Britain: National Foundation for Educational Research in England and Wales, 1972).

[122]Jon Kabat-Zinn, "Mindfulness, Stress Reduction and Healing," *Google Tech Talks*, March 8, 2007.

[123]Frederick Matthias Alexander reports incorporating these choices into his process of reeducating one's conscious control over movement and thinking as early as the late 1800s.

[124]Shian-Ling Keng, Moria Smoski and Clive Robins, "Effects of Mindfulness on Psychological Health: A Review of Empirical studies," *Clinical Psychological Review* 31 no.6 (2011): 1041-1056.

[125]Sara W. Lazar, Catherine Kerr, Rachhel H. Wasserman, and Jeremy Grey, "Meditation Experience is Associated with Increased Cortical Thickness" *Neuroreport* 16 (2005):1893-1897.

[126]Nazia Raja-Khan et al., "Mindfulness-Based Stress Reduction in Women with Overweight or Obesity: A Randomized Clinical Trial" *Obesity* 25, no. 8 (2017): 1349-1359.

[127]Arthur Ciaramicoli and Katherine Ketcham, *The Power of Empathy* (London: Piatkus Books, 2000) 113-124.

[128]Maria Konnikova, *Mastermind* (New York: Penguin Books, 2013) 254.

[129]Ibid., 255-258.

[130]Christina Bergland. "The Neuroscience of Empathy," *Psychology Today*, 10 October 2013.

[131]Jean Decety and William Ickes, T*he Social Neuroscience of Empathy* (2011) as cited in "Empathy on the Edge: Scaling and Sustaining a Human-Centered (IDEO) (human centered design)" accessed in http://cultureofempathy.com/References/Benefits/Articles.htm.

[132]Ibid.

[133]Ibid.

[134]The Freie Universitat Berlin is sponsoring a number of studies on the "neurobiology of empathy in narcissistic personality disorder," 2017 (http://www.Loc.furberlin.de/en/zentrum/forschung/negesenlossen/narzissmus).

[135]Maria Bragado and Pamela Taylor, "Empathy, Schizophrenia, and Violence: A Systematic Review," *Schizophrenic Research* 141, no. 1 (October 2012): 83-90.

[136]Norma Deitch Feshback, "Parental Empathy and Child (Mal)Adjustment," in *Empathy and Its Development*, eds. Nancy Eisenberg and Jane Strayer (New York: Cambridge University Press, 1987) 271-291.

[137]George Will, "How do we Heal our Epidemic of Loneliness?" Column in *The Washington Post*, 19 April 2020. The Sasse quotations are cited from his book, *Them: Why We Hate Each Other – And How to Heal* (New York: St. Martin's Press, 2018).

[138]"The Loneliness Epidemic," a study cited by Anthony S. Fauci, Director of the National Institute of Allergy and Infectious Diseases, and Chair of the Committee appointed by President Trump, in a press briefing on April 29, 2020.

[139]Ibid., 9.

Chapter 8

[140]Elizabeth Segal, Karen Gerdes and Alex Wagaman, "Developing the Social Empathy Index: An Exploratory Factor Analysis." *Advances in Social Work* 13, no. 3 (2012): 541-560.

[141]Charles B. Truax and Robert R. Carkhuff, *Effective Counseling and Psychotherapy* (New York: Routledge, 1976) cited in Robert Butters, A *Meta-Analysis of Empathy Training Programs for Client Populations.* (Ph.D. dissertation, The University of Utah, 2010) http://cdmbuntu.lib.utah.edu/utils/getfile/collection/etd2/id/321/filename/755.pdf

[142]Victoria Del Barrio, Anton Aluja and Luis Garcia, "Relationship between Empathy and the Big Five Personality Traits in a Sample of Spanish Adolescents." *Social Behavior and Personality* 32 (2004): 677-682.

[143]Mark H. Davis and H. Alan Oathout, "Maintenance of Satisfaction in Romantic Relationship: Empathy and Relational Competence." *Journal of Personality and Social Psychology*, 53 (1987): 397-410, cited in Robert Butters: http://cultureofempathy.com/References/Benefits/Articles.khtm

[144]Nancy Eisenberg and Paul Miller, "The Relation of Empathy to Prosocial and Related Behaviors." *Psychological Bulletin* 101 (1988): 91-119.

[145]Dianne Berg, Kimberly Lonsway and Louise Fitzgerald, "Rape Prevention Education for Men: The Effectiveness of Empathy-induction Techniques." *Journal of College Student Development* 40, no. 3 (1999): 219-234.

[146]Jean Decety and William Ickes, T*he Social Neuroscience of Empathy* (2011) as cited in "Empathy on the Edge: Scaling and Sustaining a Human-Centered (IDEO) (human centered design)" accessed in http://cultureofempathy.com/References/Benefits/Articles.htm

[147]Louis Cozolino. *The Neuroscience of Human Relationships, 2nd edition* (New York, 2014) 24.

[148]Carolyn Henry, David W. Sager, and Scott W. Plunkett, "Adolescents' Perceptions of Family System Characteristics, Parent Adolescent Dyadic Behaviors, Adolescent Qualities and Adolescent Empathy," *Family Relations* 45 (1996): 283-292.

[149]Robert Plutchik, "Integration, Differentiation, and Derivatives of Emotion," *Evolution and Cognition* 7, no. 2 (2001).

[150]Ibid.

[151]Gary Chapman, *The Five Love Languages: How to Express Heartfelt Commitment to Your Mate* (Northfield Press, 2004) and Gary Chapman and Paul White, *The Five Languages of Appreciation in the Workplace* (Northfield Press, 2011). Program for Couples in Romantic Relationships," *Family Relations* 48 (1999): 235- 242.

[152]Allen W. Barton, Ted G. Futris and Robert B. Nielsen, "Linking Financial Distress to Marital Quality: The Intermediary Roles of Demand/Withdraw and Spousal Gratitude Expressions," *Personal Relationships* 22, no. 3 (2015): 536-549.

[153]https://www.bbc.com/news/world, April 25, 2020.

[154]Ibid.

[155]Michael Gerson, "We've officially witnessed the total failure of empathy in presidential leadership," The Washington Post, https://www.washingtonpost.com/opinions, April 2, 2020.

Chapter 9

[156]David Noise, "Society Unhinged: America's Loss of Empathy," *Psychology Today,* 7 March 2016.

[157]Ibid.

[158]George Shaw, "Punishment and Reformation," *Pediatrics*, May 1975, 55, 5.

[159]Harvard University. "Winners Do Not Punish: Punishment Does Not Earn Rewards or Cooperation, Study Finds," *Science Daily*, (accessed May 7, 2017). www.sciencedaily.com/releases/2008/03/080319142358.htm.

[160] Carl R. Rogers, *On Personal Power* (New York: Delta Books, 1977) 127-129.

[161] Film available at www.strangersintownthefilm.com

[162] Carol Kusche, cited in the *Seattle News*, 20 July 2017.

[163] Brenda Salgado, *Real World Mindfulness for Beginners* (Berkeley CA: Sonoma Press, 2016) 60-61.

[164] Jeremy Rifkin, *The Empathic Civilization* (New York: Jeremy P. Tarcher/Penguin, 2009) 3

[165] Ibid., 598-9.

[166] Ibid., 601.

[167] Ibid., 605-616.

[168] Andre Tartar, "Sooner than You Think," *Bloomberg Businessweek*, 11 September 2017, 73.

[169] Steven Pinker, *Enlightenment Now: The Case for Reason, Science, Humanism, and Progress* (New York; Viking, 2018).

[170]Keith Humphries, Americans in Rural Areas More Likely to Die of Suicide, htpp://www.cdc.gov. Media/Releases/2017.

Chapter 10

[171]Joseph J. Ellis, *Founding Fathers* (New York: First Vintage Books, 2002) 5-15.

[172]Sigmund Freud, Group Psychology and the Analysis of the Ego (London: Hograrth Press, 1948) 15-21 (publication in the USA without publisher or date, ISBN #9781519492516).

[173] Carl R. Rogers, *On Personal Power* (New York: Dell Publishing Co., 1977) 237-251.

[174] Ibid., 239.

[175]William C. Cockerham, *Social Causes of Health and Disease* (Cambridge, U.K.: Polity Press, 2007) 1.

[176]Michael Marmot, *The Status Syndrome* (New York: Times Books, 2004) 2.

[177]Cockerham, 103.

[178]www.cdc.gov/violenceprevention/acestudy.

[179]Cockerham, 143.

[180]Oliver Laughland and Lauren Zanolli, "Why is Coronavirus Taking such a Deadly Toll on Black Americans?" *The Guardian*, 25 April 2020.

[181]Ibid.

[182]Ibid.

[183]"Bullying and Your Child," *Kids' Health* (Nemours Foundation, 2007).

[184]J. O'Neill, "Suicides Rise Among Middle Schoolers," *USA Today*, 16 July 2017, Section B.

[185]Ibid., 7.

[186]Ibid., 3.

[187]Christine Commaford, "The Little Black Book of Millionaire Secrets," *Forbes Magazine*, 27 August 2016.

[188]Ibid.

[189]Michelle Rodino-Colocino, "Me Too, #MeToo: Countering Cruelty with Empathy," *Communication and Critical/Cultural Studies*, 2018 (Vol. 15, No. 1, 96-106).

[190]Jo Ann Endo, "Lessons from #MeToo for Health Care Improvement," *Institute for Healthcare Improvement*, Sept 25, 2019. http://www.IHI.org.

[191]Robert Alberti and Michael Emmons. *Your Perfect Right* (San Luis Obispo, CA: Impact Publisher, 1995).

Chapter 11

[192]Leonard Zunin, *Contact: The First Four Minutes* (Los Angeles, Nash Publishing, 1972).

[193]Kim Giffin and Bobby Patton, *Fundamentals of Interpersonal Communication* (New York: Harper and Row, 1971) 120-132.

[194]Sidney Jourard, *Healthy Personality* (New York: Macmillan Publishing Co., 1974) 231.

[195]Virginia Satir, *Conjoint Family Therapy* (Palo Alto, California: Science and Behavior Books, 1967) 12.

[196]Carl R. Rogers, *On Personal Power* (New York: Dell Publishing Co., 1977) 51.

[197]Ibid., 52.

[198]Carl R. Rogers, *Becoming Partners, Marriage and Its Alternatives* (New York: Delacorte Press, 1972) 209.

[199]Erica Mondey, "Coronavirus Reshapes American Families," *Axios*, 4 April 2020.

[200]Ibid.

[201]Jourard, 239.

[202]Ibid.

[203]https://www.gottman.com/about/research/couples/

[204]John Gottman and Robert Levenson, "A Two-Factor Model for Predicting a Couple will Divorce; Exploratory Analysis Using 14-year Longitudinal Data," *Family Processes Journal.* 41.2 (2002) 83-96.

[205]Jocelyn Noveck, "With Isolation, Domestic Abuse Activists Fear 'Explosive Cocktail,'" Associated Press, April 28, 2020.

[206]Kristen Fuller, M.D., "Intimate Partner Violence and Child Abuse During COVID-19," Posted April 13, 2020.

[207]Robert Ornstein and David Sobel, *Healthy Pleasures* (Menlo Park, CA.: Addison-Wesley Publishing Co., 1989) 3-4.

[208]Ibid., 13.

[209]Ibid., 217.

[210]Debbie Gauran. "The 6 Health Benefits of Laughter," October 14, 2016, 6. www.activebea.co/Your-Health.

[211]Cited by James Gorman, "Laughter Feels So Good, Scientist Say, Because Guffaws Release Endorphins," *New York Times*, Sept 14, 2011, A14.

[212]Markhan Heid. "You Asked: Does Laughing Have Real Health Benefits?" *Time*, 19 November 2014, 16-18.

[213]Ibid.

[214]Sarah Pressman and Tara Kraft, Psychologists at the University of Kansas, cited in Brenda Salgordo, *Real World Mindfulness for Beginners* (Berkeley, CA: Sonoma Press, 2016) 40.

[215]Ornstein and Sobel, Ibid., 4.

[216]Ibid., 5.

[217]Ibid.

[218]Teresa Seeman and Eileen Crimmins, "Social Environment Effects on Health and Aging," *Annals of the New York Academy of Science*, 954, December, 2001

Chapter 12

[219]https://www.MEDIFIND.com/news/post/problems-us-healthcare-system, October 15, 2021.

[220]Ibid.

[221]Mary Gerisch, "Health Care as a Human Right", https://www.americanbar.org/groups/crsj/publications/human_rights_magazine October, 2021

[222]National Center for Health Statistics. Center for Disease Control and Prevention, 2 July, 2021 Report.

[223]https://www.bloomberg.com/news/articles /2021-07-21/covid-19-takes-dramatic-toll-on-u-s-life-expectancy

[224]Ibid.

[225]Kathleen Parker, "Crisis Calls for Unity and Optimism: We Have Little of Either," *The Washington Post*, 9 May 2020.

[226]Alex Korb, *The Upward Spiral* (Oakland, CA: New Harbinger Publications, Inc., 2015) 64-74.

[227]Jonathan W. Page, *NeuroCop* (Lawrence, KS: World is Round, LLC Press, 2015).

[228]Malcolm Gladwell, *Blink: The Power of Thinking Without Thinking* (New York: Little, Brown, and Company, 2007).

[229]Charles Duhigg, *The Power of Habit* (New York: Random House Trade Paperback Edition, 2014) 92.

[230]Ibid., 93.

[231]Barbara Given, *Teaching to the Brain's Natural Learning Systems* (Alexandria, VA.: Assoc. for Supervision and Curriculum Development, 2002) 9. Lesson plans are given to help develop reflective thinking.

[232]Ibid., 14.

[233]This analysis is suggested by Gavin DeBecker, *Fear Less* (New York: Little, Brown and Company) 2002.

[234]Geshe Kelsang Gyatso, *Transform Your Life: A Blissful Journey* (New York: Tharpa Publications, 2015).

Chapter 13

[235]Mark Knapp, *Social Intercourse: From Greeting to Goodbye* (Boston: Allyn and Bacon, 1978).

[236]Adam Gazzaley and Larry D. Posen. *The Distracted Mind: Ancient Brains in a High-tech World* (Cambridge, MA: MIT Press, 2016).

[237]Matthew McKay and Patrick Fanning, *Self-Esteem* (New York: MJF Books, 2000) 289-285.

[238]Mary Gordon, *The Roots of Empathy* (New York: Thomas Allen Publishers, 2009).

[239]Ibid., 4-5.

[240]Michael Weitzman, cited in Tiffany Sharples, "A User's Guide to Good Health at Every Age," *Time*, 22 June 2009, 86.

[241]Bella M. DePaulo, *Singled Out: How Singles Are Stereotyped, Stigmatized, and Ignored, and Still Live Happily Ever After* (New York: St. Martins Griffin, 2007).

[242]Ibid.

[243]Ibid.

[244]Bella M. DePaulo, *How We Live Now: Redefining Home and Family in the 21st Century* (Hillsboro, OR: Atria Books/Beyond Words, 2015).

[245]Cheryl M. Hamilton, *Communicating for Results: A Guide for Business and the Professions, 11th Ed.* (New York: Wadsworth, 2018), and Kelly M. Quintanilla and Shawn T. Wahl, *Business and Professional Excellence: Keys for Workplace Excellence, 4th Ed.* (Sage Publications, Incorporated, 2019).

[246]*The US Army Leadership Field Manual No. 22-100* (New York: McGraw-Hill, 2004).

[247]Ibid., 115.

[248]Prudence Gourguechon, "Is Trump Mentally Fit to be President? Let's Consult the U.S. Army's Field Manual on Leadership." *Los Angeles Times*, 16 June 2017.

[249]*Army Leadership Field Manual*, 34.

[250]Ibid.

[251]Ibid., 175.

Chapter 14

[252]Sydney M. Jourard, *Healthy Personality* (New York: Macmillan Publishing Co., 1974) 180.

[253]Adapted with permission from Jack Gibb, "Defensive Communication," *Journal of Communication* 11, 3 (1961): 142-148.

[254]Sidney Blumenthal, "Trump's Increasingly Weird Attempts to Compare Himself to Lincoln," *The New Yorker*, 24 October 2019

[255]Danielle Bassett, "How the Brain's Wiring Leads to Cognitive Control," *Nature Communications* 10, October 6, 2015, 38-41

[256]Max Stendahl, "Boston's Akili says video game helped children with ADHD in landmark study," *Boston Business Journal*, 4 December 2017.

[257]Cited by D. Baer, "Where Will Happens in the Brain," *New York Magazine*, 6 January 2017, 4-6.

[258]Ibid.

[259]Jonathan W. Page, *NeuroCop.* (Lawrence, Kansas: World is Round, LLC, 2015).

[260]Ibid., 127.

[261]Kevin Rector. "Baltimore Recruits Receive Cognitive Training to Better Handle Stress," *The Baltimore Sun*, 5 August 2016, 6.

[262]Jonathan W. Page, "How TAC-Talk Can Prevent Unintended Discharges," PoliceOne.com News, 13 March 2015. https://policeone.com/Officer-Safety/articles/8547380

[263]Ibid.

[264]Ibid.

[265]Ibid., 128-132.

[266]Robert Wright, "The Meditation Cure," *The Wall Street Journal*, 29-30 July 2017.

[267]Brenda Salgado, *Real World Mindfulness for Beginners* (Berkeley, CA: Sonoma Press, 2016) 17.

[268]Ben Rogers and Emily Robinson, *The Benefits of Community Engagement. A Review of Evidence* (London: Active Citizenship Centre, 2004).

[269]Glenn Laverack, *Health Promotion Practice: Power and Empowerment* (London, Sage Publishing, 2014) 36-40.

[270]Nina Wallerstein, *What is the Evidence on Effectiveness of Empowerment to Improve Health*, a Report from the Health Evidence Network, 2006.

[271]Michael Sherman, *Heavens on Earth* (New York: Henry Holt and Company, 2018) 79-80.

Other books by Bobby R. Patton

Fundamentals of Interpersonal Communication
(with Kim Giffin).

Basic Readings in Interpersonal Communication
(with Kim Giffin).

Problem-Solving Group Interaction
(with Kim Giffin).

Living Together...Female/Male Communication
(with Bonnie Ritter Patton).

Interpersonal Communication in Action
(with Kim Giffin).

Interpersonal Communication in Nursing
(with Kim Giffin and Bonnie Duldt).

Responsible Public Speaking
(with Kim Giffin and Wil Linkugel).

Personal Communication in Human Relations
(with Kim Giffin, edited by Carl Rogers and William Colson).

Decision-Making Group Interaction: Achieving Quality
(with Timothy M. Downs)

CPSIA information can be obtained
at www.ICGtesting.com
Printed in the USA
LVHW050620100123
736833LV00008B/419